200,000,000 GUINEA PIGS

Other Books by *JOHN G. FULLER*

THE GENTLEMEN CONSPIRATORS
THE MONEY CHANGERS
INCIDENT AT EXETER
INTERRUPTED JOURNEY
THE DAY OF ST. ANTHONY'S FIRE
THE GREAT SOUL TRIAL

200,000,000 Guinea Pigs

NEW DANGERS IN EVERYDAY FOODS, DRUGS, AND COSMETICS

by John G. Fuller

G. P. Putnam's Sons, New York

Copyright © 1972 by John G. Fuller

SBN: 399-11000-3
Library of Congress Catalog Card Number: 72-79521
PRINTED IN THE UNITED STATES OF AMERICA

To
Arthur Kallet and F. J. Schlink,
whose book 100,000,000 Guinea Pigs *pioneered*
in the work of exposing those who put
profit ahead of human values and safety,
when the country's population was half
the size it is now
and
To P. E., who must
remain anonymous

Contents

Introduction

IN 1933, the book *100,000,000 Guinea Pigs*, by Arthur Kallet and F. J. Schlink, shocked and awakened the country to the dangers in everyday foods, drugs, and cosmetics.

The book took a cold, angry look at the hazards and inadequacies of such things as prescription drugs, toothpastes, mouthwashes, cereals, germicides, meats, food additives, lead poisoning, cosmetics, aspirin, hair dyes, cold remedies, over-the-counter drugs, alleged medical devices, wild and irresponsible advertising claims, and the lack of enforcement of protective regulations by government agencies.

At about the same time, the Food and Drug Administration made it known that the original, hoary Food and Drug Act of 1906, as advanced as it was for its day, needed major surgery to bring it up to date.

With *100,000,000 Guinea Pigs* awakening the indifferent and inattentive consumer of the thirties, a long battle shaped up in Congress for more sensible legislation to protect the public from glaring abuses imposed on it by manufacturers. Characteristically, many large pharmaceutical and grocery corporations fought the proposed consumer legislation with every mortar, pestle, and meat cleaver at their command.

100,000,000 Guinea Pigs sparked a rising wave of consumer indignation. It played an important role in the eventual passage of the 1938 Food, Drug, and Cosmetic Act. But if there is anything that history shows us about consumerism, it is

that it takes a major catastrophe to carry legal and enforcement action over the hump of lethargy and resistance.

The 1938 law sprang from the fumes of the tall, dark bottles labeled ELIXIR SULFANILAMIDE. A chemist of the S. E.
Massengill Company managed to mix a pharmaceutical
cocktail with deadly ethylene glycol. No testing for safety of
new drugs was required then, and over 100 innocent people
promptly died. As a result, the new legislation was swept in
over few objections, and these came, of course, from certain
pharmaceutical, cosmetic, and grocery houses.

If the sulfa tragedy completed the attack against lethargy,
Kallet and Schlink's book softened the ground for it. But
there was no way for the authors to predict at that time what
the future held in store for food, drugs, and cosmetics—to say
nothing of health devices, general household hazards, lethal
toys, and environmental dangers affecting everything and everyone.

Today, nearly forty years later, the situation is worse, not
better. Every new advance seems to have brought with it a
more than equal share of danger. New hazards are more sub-
tle, more sophisticated, more deadly than those of the less
regulated days of the early thirties.

Time bombs are ticking today in several dark corners.
Warnings of experts have been and are going unheeded. A
small group of dedicated people in government service, in
Congress, in consumer groups, as well as some independent
citizens, are attempting to combat the abuses imposed by
those in industry who glaringly put profit ahead of social
welfare at the expense of the consumer and in some cases at
his mortal peril. It is 1933 all over again—multiplied by logarithms. The difference is only a matter of form.

This is not a book on the broad expanse of the new consumer movement. This is a book about consumer *danger*.
Pricing and quality of goods and services are important—but
they are secondary. As one FDA official wryly commented:
*"I've been cheated and I've been poisoned, and believe me, cheated is
better."*

The life or death of the consumer comes first. The consumer population is no longer 100,000,000. There are twice that number—200,000,000 guinea pigs today—far too many to be caged, tagged, fed, and drugged for the sake of exploitative profit.

J. G. F.

Westport, Conn.

If there is to be an end to the wholesale poisoning of the public by food and drug manufacturers, the relationship of enforcement officials to both the manufacturers and the public must be clearly understood and continually in plain view.

—Arthur Kallet and F. J. Schlink,
in *100,000,000 GUINEA PIGS*

200,000,000 GUINEA PIGS

1

Consumer Roulette

IT IS an ordinary, routine shopping day.

You are rolling your supermarket cart toward a bewildering maze of stuffed and brightly colored shelves, where a fairyland of food supplies is waiting for you. The check-out registers are thumping metallically behind you, and a white-coated stock man is punching out the 2/41 price stamp on a case of Campbell's Manhandler soup, in counterrhythm to the cash register.

You are vaguely familiar with the Food and Drug Administration, the Federal Trade Commission, the Department of Agriculture, and several other government agencies that have been looking after your interests as a shopper for a good many years, and there is considerable comfort in that thought. You believe that they are doing a lot of your worrying for you.

You know, for instance, that cyclamates are no longer lurking in your diet cola drinks, but there's a possibility you don't know there is a considerable amount of caffeine in them. There's no reason why anyone who wants to drink caffeine should not have it, but parents who aren't too keen on having their young children surfeited with the drug might at least want to know about it from the label. There is considerable evidence about the relationship of caffeine intake to heart disease. For a second thought, you might also wonder why it took so long to get cyclamates off the market. And what about saccharin as the new diet drink delight? Will it come out unscathed from the new, penetrating studies that are being conducted on it by the National Academy of Sciences?

The laws and regulations of the Food and Drug Administration form the principal bulwark against untoward contamination of your food. They have improved over the years. Just how adequately the understaffed and underbudgeted agency can *enforce* these laws is open to question—even if a new, independent agency is set up, as Congress proposed in June, 1972.

Under the latest act, FDA inspectors and scientists are concerned with unsafe food additives; pesticide residues; improper food packaging; cancer-producing, or carcinogenic, food coloring; filthy, putrid, or decomposed foods; misleading labels and "slack-fill" packages swollen by corrugated padding; rat and mouse hairs and excreta; whole insects; insect parts and excreta; maggots; larvae and parasitic worms; human excreta and sewage pollution; transportation accidents causing foods to be insect-infested; moldy food; foods contaminated by ore concentrates or insecticides; salmonella and botulism poisoning; overfumigation; specific excreta of beetles, moths, bats, chickens, goats, and camels.

The FDA is trying to do your worrying for you about underprocessing, defective containers, preservatives, and decomposed or overpreserved fish—the kind that might have a repulsive form of parasite-producing cysts and puslike material in their flesh.

Beyond this, there is FDA concern about clams harboring the bacterium *Gonyaulax catenella*; bacteria spoilage; mercury and other poisonous metals; rancidity; the deadly aflatoxin often found in nuts; natural hydrocyanic acid—the list goes on. The problems with cosmetics, over-the-counter drugs, prescription drugs, herbicides, and insecticides are equally imposing.

There is a poster hanging on the walls of several FDA offices, an ironic reminder of the problems some of the overworked staff have faced over a recent twelve-month period. It is a long strip of poster paper that reads:

TUNA FISH

SWORDFISH

KINGFISH

BREAKABLE RATTLES

LOUD TOY GUNS

TOY DARTS

DANGEROUS DOLLS; STUFFED ANIMALS

SQUEAKERS, NOISEMAKERS

CYCLAMATES

ORINASE DIABETES PILLS

SALT AND MSG IN BABY FOOD

THYROID-AMPHETAMINE DIET PILLS

DDT

PARATHION

2,4,5-T WEED KILLER

SHELL OIL CO. NO-PEST STRIPS

RELAXACISORS

SACCHARIN

BIRTH CONTROL PILLS

C-QUENS ORAL CONTRACEPTIVES

PROVEST ORAL CONTRACEPTIVES

UNSAFE WATER SUPPLIES

BROMINATED VEGETABLE OILS

MICROWAVE OVENS

NTA IN DETERGENTS

2,4-TDA IN HAIR DYE

COSMETICS CONTAINING MERCURY

BUBBLE CLUB FUN BATH

MR. BUBBLE

MEXICAN AND OTHER POTTERY CONTAINING LEAD

INDIAN NECKLACES MADE OF POISON BEANS

28 CONTAMINATED COSMETICS

696 INEFFECTIVE OR CONTAMINATED DRUGS

KRAFT CHEESE CONTAINING PESTICIDE

SPICE OF LIFE MEAT TENDERIZER

COUNTRY TAVERN MEAT TENDERIZER

HOLLYWOOD MILK SHAKE CANDY BARS

PIZZA CONTAINING BOTULISM

LIPTON SOUP MIX CONTAINING SALMONELLA

Symbolizing the number of groans a conscientious FDA staff man might encounter in his daily routine, the poster covers only a fraction of the headaches that pour into the offices of the administration all over the country each day. As a partial reminder, the poster might well be used as a negative shopping list, although many of these particular problems have now been solved. Those that have been solved will find many substitutes ready to take their places.

The mercury problem in tuna and swordfish is destined to persist, although a temporary if tenuous tolerance of .05 parts per million has been set by the FDA. The tuna on the shelves is under this limit, but swordfish has been found to exceed it by several times. The fact is that no one really knows what the safe limit is.

Breakable rattles, loud toy guns that can damage hearing, toy darts, dangerous dolls, stuffed animals, squeakers, and noisemakers are constantly appearing and disappearing from the market. The price of child safety is constant parental alertness.

The cyclamate story is still important. It may well reflect the fate of many hidden hazards in other food additives that are now regarded as safe. It also represents a constant pattern of callous disregard of industry toward public safety. If there is one rule, one axiom, one truism that has become apparent over the years, it is that industry will never regulate itself, in spite of all its protestations to the contrary. Whether Congress sets up a new agency to replace the FDA or not will have little effect.

Orinase diabetes pills, next on the poster listing these FDA headaches, are produced by the large, "ethical" pharmaceutical house Upjohn. The drug was the subject of a study beginning in 1960 and culminating in 1969. The conclusion was that the pills were not only less effective than diet control or insulin, but that test groups which took the drug showed a greater death rate compared to control groups. It took until March, 1970, for the FDA warnings to be issued. Ironically, an Upjohn scientist had shortly before written a paper about the drug in the prestigious *Journal of the American Medical Association* for a patently obvious reason: to persuade prescribing doctors that non-brand-name, or generic, drugs could not be depended on. The irony lay not only in the later warnings about the safety of Orinase. The Upjohn scientist had contrived his own nonmarketed generic version of the drug, thus setting up a straw man. He avoided any mention that some statistics have shown that cheaper generic drugs actually have a better track record for safety and efficacy than the big-brand-name equivalents.

Salt in baby food has been subjected to a series of hard, tough looks by scientists, as has another additive, MSG (monosodium glutamate), principally marketed as Accent. Both had been added to baby foods so that the mother would find it more palatable when she pretasted it. Infants have little, if any, sense of taste. There is considerable scientific opinion that the use of too much salt by infants in their formative years creates an unnecessary dependency on excessive quantities to the eventual detriment of their health. Chinese, for instance, have been known to commit suicide by eating a cup of salt. Although the risk in using MSG as a flavor enhancer in adult foods is thought to be small, it has produced defects in the brains and retinas of newborn animals.

From the countrywide point of view, the Food and Drug Administration attempts to throw up a thin shield of protection between us and the hazards that are multiplying daily in the headlong rush for profits by the food, drug, and other manufacturers.

As the principal guardian of choice on the national scene, the FDA has been provided by the White House and the Bureau of the Budget with an annual funding roughly equivalent to the amount furnished the Los Angeles County Sheriff's Office for its operations. The recent $83,000,000 budget of the FDA tries to regulate a heavily profit-minded food industry nearly 1,600 times its size in dollar volume, a drug industry some 50 times its size, and a cosmetic industry also 50 times its size. The sales volume of the Great Atlantic & Pacific Tea Company alone is 72 times the FDA's budget.

The FDA staff of some 4,500 employees is no better or worse than any average cross section of employable people. Some are intense, dedicated, well trained, and competent. Many are less than that. Others are flatly incompetent. On balance, the sense of dedication seems to be dominant among the professional staff. The big problem arises with the top-level officials. These are political appointees who have shown over the years a consistent pattern of favoring big industry over the consumer when it comes to critical issues. There is little evidence that this trend is changing or will change even with a new form of agency.

Assume, though, for a moment at least, that the policy-making officials are not at all influenced by the gargantuan lobbyists of the trade associations and big-industry pressure. How adequate would the FDA's protection be?

Its responsibilities are staggering. It not only has to cope with the way foods and drugs are manufactured. It must try to control the frequent outbreaks of salmonella and staphylococcus poisonings, botulism threats, and the major worldwide concern about chemical food additives. It must try to set and patrol legal tolerances for pesticide residues, mercury pollution, and the cleanliness of foods.

It must conduct hearings, fight court battles, approve or disapprove new drug applications, arrange for recalls of some drugs or foods—or seize them when the producer involved fails to cooperate. It must inspect thousands of tons of imported foods and drugs, to say nothing of offering a clearing house for poison control centers.

To keep an eye on all this frenetic activity, it has a force of some 650 inspectors, less than half the size of the Newark, New Jersey, uniformed police force.

In spite of a considerable amount of dedication to the job by this force, the consumer cannot feel altogether comfortable in this situation. The FDA's Lilliputian budget has not at all been helped by President Richard Nixon, who has consistently instructed the Bureau of the Budget to lower the amounts appropriated by Congress for the critical life-and-death functions of the FDA. In one area of FDA activity, Congress appropriated $691,000. The President requested that this sum be entirely eliminated.

Safety protection is stretched to the thinnest film imaginable in all areas of responsibility by sheer lack of manpower and funds. Take, for instance, the imports of manufactured dairy products. FDA inspectors have their hands full in inspecting only 4 percent of the material. But they found that 12 percent of everything seized was insanitary or adulterated.

While the FDA can often be criticized for overstating its capacity for protecting the consumer, many of the staff executives are frank to admit the limitations they work under.

Many consumers think that all foods on the market are in compliance with all FDA food regulations. Maurice Kinslow, chairman of an FDA study group, who is in a position to know about this with great accuracy, states firmly: "If consumers believe that all food is in compliance, they are not justified in believing that."

Charles C. Johnson, a well-known Public Health Service

administrator, goes a step further. "We know that what the public thinks is happening and what we are able to produce just isn't always the same."

Congressmen and Senators are intensely alert to the consumer's complaints today. Consumers are not quite in a position today where they merely trouble a deaf heaven with their bootless cries. They may even get action.

The solution to the pesticide residues that saturate food products promises to remain outside the capacity of both Congress and the regulatory agencies. There are about 900 different pesticide compounds. Gas chromatography tests can identify only about 60 of them. Others require more lengthy testing. Naturally, it is impossible for the FDA to examine every interstate shipment of food in the country, and it has no jurisdiction at all over locally distributed foods. The attempt now is to examine the pesticide that clings to foods in about 1 percent of the shipments that cross state lines. While the average levels of the residues seem to be within limits that are recognized as acceptable, there is still the question about the overenthusiastic sprayer who douses his crops in an uneven way, with overdoses on some parts and none on others. The consumer who gets the overloaded dose has small comfort in learning that this particular crop had an *average* safe level.

It is at this point that the persistent, inescapable drumbeat comes in: The large agricultural interests and their trade associations are fighting to prevent any restrictions on their use of pesticides and herbicides that might cut down profits. Only minor effects on food production would be felt in this country if pesticide use was reduced up to 80 percent, according to Barry Commoner, of Washington University, St. Louis. About the kindest thing you could say about their attitude is that it is shortsighted.

The two most prominent swords of Damocles that hang over the FDA are future incidents that may repeat the Elixir of Sulfanilamide disaster of 1937 and the thalidomide tragedy of 1962. This sedative drug, new at the time, resulted in thousands of newborn babies coming into the world without limbs or with other grotesque defects. Dr. Frances O. Kelsey, an FDA medical officer, stubbornly refused to accept the new drug application for thalidomide, in spite of the pressure put on her by the William S. Merrell Company, a major pharmaceutical firm and subsidiary of Vick Chemical. In doing so, she not only prevented the mass deformities that shook Europe, where the drug had been distributed, but she brought action to a sluggish Congress to pass the 1962 Kefauver-Harris amendments to the 1938 Food, Drug, and Cosmetic Act. These were the first major amendments since the 1930's. For the first time, prescription drugs would now have to be proved not only safe but at least as effective as a sugar pill. All through the years, from 1938 to 1962, it was not necessary for the manufacturer to prove that his drug would do what he claimed it would do.

But the evolution in the life-or-death consumer protection areas is painfully slow. In the halls of Congress and the FDA, there is a feeling that somewhere there have got to be new disasters brewing that will break suddenly on the scene, just as with the sulfanilamide and thalidomide tragedies. Laws are passed that add to the responsibilities of the Food and Drug Administration, but the Bureau of the Budget has failed to allocate any realistic amounts to provide for their enforcement. For instance, not a single dime was provided when the 1968 Fair Packaging and Labelling Act was enacted.

One senior FDA official said: "There are two definite areas right now, to say nothing of others, that are clearly time bombs. One is cosmetics, where we are still operating under the old 1938 laws, and nothing has been changed since. The other is in therapeutic devices—everything from weight reduction gimmicks to the Relaxacisor. We have just now got that off the market, after 10 years of litigation. There are dozens of devices around right now, and nobody really knows what the hell they are, and what damage they can do. To name just one, we don't know what these blow-up weight reducers do. None of them are required to show any pretesting or standards before they hit the market. The only way we can get at them is through the courts—and that can take years."

The consumer often reads about FDA "recalls" and FDA "seizures." Contrary to public opinion, there is no rule that forces a manufacturer to recall a defective or dangerous product outside of court action. What the FDA has to depend on is the threat of publicity, which is fortunately remarkably effective in bringing about a "voluntary" withdrawal of the product from the dealers' shelves.

Seizures, in contrast to recalls, can be made on any food, drug, device, or cosmetic that is adulterated or misbranded. This procedure stands as a threat to the manufacturer who refuses to cooperate with a voluntary recall. But seizures must be made of only one shipment at a time, a long, expensive process that involves moving through the U.S. District Courts.

These two basic tools are put into effect constantly by FDA enforcement officers. However, the products that should have been seized or recalled are still uncounted. There were 600 seizures and 1,427 recalls in 1970. If the FDA had an adequate enforcement staff, the figure would surely be considerably greater. Dr. Charles C. Edwards, recent FDA Commissioner, said bluntly: "I am astounded, having come from industry, and particularly realizing the fact that we regulate industries that have a net worth of something in the neighborhood of $200 billion to $300 billion, that we are trying to do this job on a budget of $70 million or $80 million. It just can't be done adequately in my judgment."

There are many areas that need urgent FDA attention. Teratogenicity—the damage that can be passed on to newborn children, as in the thalidomide case—is a very real threat to the consumer. He eats foods and takes drugs with chemicals and additives with long-term effects no scientist can predict. And carcinogenicity—the capacity to induce cancer—can lurk in many formerly unsuspected chemicals and additives. Add to these the third horseman of the consumer apocalypse, mutagenicity, which is the capacity of causing changes that can continue forever in the germ plasm, and you have a grim scene. It is made worse by the manufacturers who heedlessly load their foods, drugs, and cosmetics with a plethora of additives for the sake of making their products more salable and profitable. As one Congressional investigator stated with firm conviction: "1984 is *here!*"

Congressman L. H. Fountain, a steadfast crusader in attempting to stem the tide of chemical acrobatics the manufacturers are perpetrating, said in regard to one dangerous drug: "I feel compelled to express my own personal concern over FDA's lack of vigor in protecting the public, and especially children, against the continued marketing of a drug . . . which could result in irreparable harm and even death." The consumer can be both wary and worried, regardless of whether the fault lies in FDA inefficiency or lack of staff or both.

There is no question that the FDA is overloaded and that this factor alone is enough to chill the bones of perceptive and intelligent consumers. But almost worse than that is the force and power of the lobbyists, corporations, and trade associations that attempt to block any important action by the agency. As Dr. Herbert Ley, a former FDA Commissioner, said: "I am under constant, tremendous and sometimes unmerciful pressure from the drug industry." Regarding a most important National Academy of Sciences review of the effectiveness of all drugs marketed during the 1938–62 period, he said: "It is now apparent that the resistance of industry is going to be both intense and prolonged."

For the consumer, there are two dragons to slay: the venality of the giant, profit-minded food, drug, and cosmetic industries, and a giant lack of resources in the FDA. Or as Dr. Ley summed it up: "Our zeal is high. To quote the Scriptures, the spirit is willing, but sometimes the body is weak . . . we do not have enough hands to really pursue the task as promptly and effectively as we would like to."

Meanwhile, 200,000,000 guinea pigs sit, and wait, and go about their daily shopping, hoping and often wistfully believing that something is being done.

2

One Brief Slice of Time

THE CONSUMER'S stake in the enormous crap game that is being played daily with his life and well-being by the profit-oriented, lobby-minded industries can be most graphically pictured by taking a close look at a sample period of activity over a selected slice of time. The first half of 1971 is a good illustration.

When 1971 was ushered in with the usual bells, horns, and migraines, the currents where the consumer's life and safety were concerned were boiling like white water in a chain of rapids. It was no different from any other time period, really. The details during the first few months of 1971 will illustrate what is going on at the moment you are reading this book, or before, or probably years after. The conditions are bound to prevail unless the consumer becomes more awake, forces authorities to take realistic action, and protests that he no longer has a fondness for remaining a guinea pig.

The year 1971, as our sample, began with a scene that could be described charitably as chaotic as far as the consumer was concerned. The dramatis personae were principally the Food and Drug Administration, the Congressional watchdog committees, the food and drug trade associations, the manufacturers themselves, an indifferent Nixon administration, the Federal Trade Commission, the National Academy of Sciences, and the many other federal, state, and municipal organizations charged with the heroic attempt of protecting the protagonist of the drama—the bewildered and vulnerable consumer.

The new year 1971 inherited several echoes from the previous one. In Georgia, the president of the firm Yates and Wheeler, Inc., pleaded guilty to the charges that he had made an interstate shipment of cabbages that were over-soaked with the pesticide chemical toxaphene. He was slapped on the wrist with a $100 fine and placed on probation for five years.

Two of the great "ethical" drug houses, Merck, Sharp & Dohme and a subsidiary of the Sterling Drug Company found themselves facing FDA withdrawal of approval of their bronchial inhalers. They were judged to be ineffective in combating asthma, emphysema, and bronchitis.

Eli Lilly and Company and the Upjohn Company, two other prestigious giants of the drug industry, finally agreed to take the oral contraceptive C-Quens and Provest off the market. Beagle dogs tested with the drugs began showing up with breast nodules. Components in the drugs are not found in other oral contraceptives, but there is the nagging wonder as to why Lilly and Upjohn didn't find all this out *before* they put their products on the market.

Stokely-Van Camp, a major foodstuffs manufacturer, found its canned peach slices, pear halves, and plums seized by the FDA on mislabeling charges.

U.S. Plywood, during the previous year, was smarting under a notice of judgment and seizure action by the FDA on its Weldwood contact cement product for not putting adequate warning on the labels of this extremely flammable product.

In Baltimore, the Potomac Creamery Company finally accepted a permanent injunction on on interstate shipment of its nonfat dry milk alleged by the FDA to be riddled with salmonella microorganisms. The preliminary injunction had been filed in 1967. In the meantime, the product enjoyed shelf space on the market.

In Boston, a consumer was astute enough to report to the local FDA office the sale by a Boston department store of necklaces made from the deadly imported jequirity bean. A nervous chew on a necklace is not an uncommon practice, and it would take very few nibbles before the wearer would topple over in a fatal coma.

In Denver, an FDA inspector just *happened* to notice an exterminator at work in a Montana noodle manufacturer's plant. The exterminator was using the dangerous pesticide chlordane. Later tests showed that the noodles were far off-limits for chlordane residues. But worse than that, the new batches of noodles manufactured to replace the recalled shipments also were coated with chlordane. The firm was forced to stop all manufacturing at this plant.

In Minneapolis, a mother treated her college-age daughter to a going-away party and rustled up some popcorn for the festivities. She canceled this part of the menu when she discovered, in her own words, "frantic little worms wriggling around in the hot oil." The FDA arranged immediately for the voluntary destruction of some $200 worth of packaged popcorn.

In New York, FDA inspectors found that a three-year-old child had chewed on the painted red handle of a toy broom, and the child's blood tests proved to have 30 parts per million lead level. Scrapings from the broom had about 25,000 parts per million, and the child came down with serious lead poisoning.

Many sacrosanct drugs and dentifrices were singled out by the FDA to be withdrawn from the market. They included Cēpacol Mouthwash and Gargle, Colgate Dental Cream with Gardol, Lederle's Achromycin Troches, Squibb's Mysteclin Pediatric Drops, Pepsodent Antiseptic Mouthwash, Amm-i-Dent toothpaste and powder, Kolynos Fluoride Toothpaste, Micrin Oral Antiseptic, Winthrop's Neo-Synephrine-Sulfathiazolate Nose Drops, and literally scores of other products by blue-chip companies such as Wyeth, Warner-Chilcott, Upjohn, Armour Pharmaceutical, Merck, Sharp & Dohme, Squibb, Abbott, Lilly, Johnson & Johnson, Parke-Davis, Bristol, CIBA, and others. The list reads like an industrial social register. The companies immediately began to assemble their heavy legal artillery to fight the ban.

Some of the products have already been removed from the market; others are still there on pending actions to contest the FDA's contention that "there is a lack of substantial evidence of effectiveness or an unfavorable benefit-to-risk ratio."

For the consumer, this phrase "benefit-to-risk ratio" is most critical, and it is probably the most often repeated phrase whenever any action is considered by the FDA or in weighing its decisions.

It *is* critical. For a patient suffering from terminal cancer, a drug might have serious dangers but would still be worth trying if there were a fragment of a chance that it might be effective. The possible benefits might outweigh the serious risks. On the other hand, a remedy for the possible relief of cold symptoms must have practically no risk whatever, or else it could be worse than the cold itself. Safety and effectiveness go hand in hand; there is practically no separation.

Other echoes ringing in FDA ears in 1971 came from the recently inherited responsibilities imposed on the agency by the Child Protection and Toy Safety Act, which became effective in 1970. Toys that offered the possibility of electric shocks, mechanical hazards, burns, or strangulation possibilities were beginning to get a severe going over *for the first time* under FDA auspices.

The targets selected for the first survey included the dolls, infant toys, and battery-operated novelty toys of the Ideal Toy Company, the woodburning outfits and melting kits of Mattel, Inc., the housekeeping and battery-operated toys of Remco Industries, the hobby horses and infant vehicles of Hasbro Industries—many of which have been saturating the television air waves *ad nauseam*. There are dozens of others on the proposed survey list that had been happily on the market for considerable time with no real knowledge on the part of the consumer as to whether they were safe or not.

Some of the most obvious hazardous toys were immediate targets for banning for child use, such as the lethal lawn

darts of Hasbro Industries and the R. B. Jarts Company,
darts that a Watusi chieftain would be proud to carry to battle.

The stuffed toy cats and animal heads sold by the elegant
Georg Jensen, Inc., were found to have enchanting eyes, but
they were easily removable to reveal long, sharp metal pins
to dim the affections of a child who poked one in his own eye
or face. A long succession of rubber squeaker toys of various
manufacturers were found to have easily removable squeaker
buttons that could change a child's squeal of delight to a
scream of anguish when it caught in his windpipe. Prizewin-
ners contending for a mythical Thoughtless Manufacturer of
the Week award included the Jiggly rattle of the Bomar
Company, with a breakable handle that exposed sharp metal
protrusions; the Moody Doll from Holiday Fair, Inc., with
pins and a long spike in the neck; the Musical Merry-Go-
Round Canelon from F. W. Woolworth, with metal spikes
and a pasteboard exterior; and sharp-pointed arrow archery
sets from Bear Archery Company and Fleetwood Archery,
labeled for use by children up to seven and eight years old,
respectively.

Nor were the FDA inspectors particularly enchanted with
the Weiner Whistle of the Oscar Mayer Company, just $2\frac{1}{N}$
inches long, attached to each package of Oscar Mayer hot
dogs and convenient enough in size to fit snugly in the gullet
of a small child.

As 1971 began in earnest, recalls were no more startling
than in any other period of the monotonous history of recalls.
Lederle Labs Division of American Cyanamid was reported
during the week of January 7 in a recall of all lots of its shipments of Achromycin nasal suspension product, as well as its
Achromycin Pharynjets. Also under recall by the same blue-
chip company were many of its other Achromycin products
and its Gevramet Geriatric Elixir.

During the same week, other recalls included foods of
many types, from Peanut Patties for rodent infestation to
Monark Egg Corporation's Food Egg Mix for salmonella
contamination. Land O' Lakes joined the recall parade

when its Co-op Powdered Nonfat Instant Dry Milk fortified with vitamins A and D was found to have "faulty disintegration." About 200,000 pounds were withdrawn from the market.

Johnson & Johnson, not at all happy about the FDA slings and arrows directed at its favorite mouthwash, Micrin, found itself forced to withdraw its sterile eye pads in $3\frac{3}{4}$-inch boxes, twelve to a box, when it was discovered that they were more contaminated than they were sterile.

The renowned Scripto company, noted for its pens and profits, went about the long process of recalling some fifty gross of its sterile disposable surgical skin-marking pens when it was discovered that they were definitely not sterile.

But all this was reported over the period of only one week. Through the rest of the month over twenty products were recalled, including everything from Miles Laboratories' Nysta-Cort $\frac{1}{2}$% lotion, to the Great Atlantic and Pacific Tea Company's frozen swordfish, ominously loaded with highly significant mercury levels, as all swordfish were found to be.

Dr. Charles Edwards, the recently appointed Commissioner of the FDA, was turning his attention not only to the myriad problems within his organization but toward placating the sullen if not mutinous grumbles of the large and impatient consumer movements.

He explained in a speech to the Consumer Federation in January, 1971, that the FDA's prime mandate from Congress was administering regulations and that this was relatively simple. (He did not, however, elaborate on how 650 field inspectors could, with or without track shoes, cover the vast and staggering areas they were assigned to cover.) He explained that the mobilization of scientific evidence and informed scientific opinion was an exceedingly complex matter. "This fact," he said, "is often lost to those not intimately familiar with FDA operations. Everybody seems to know that we are a regulatory agency concerned with consumer protection. *Not* everybody is aware that we are also a *scientific* agency."

With the appointment of Malcolm W. Jensen as director

of the Bureau of Product Safety in early 1971, industry began worrying about where it stood in this area. As usual, it was caught shorthanded. Practically no concerted effort had been made in the private sector to attempt to set up voluntary safety standards, just as the auto industry had done practically nothing until Ralph Nader came along. Jensen's indications that he might turn his attention toward bicycles, rotary lawn mowers, temperatures for floor furnaces, and surface temperatures for ranges and incinerators, among other things, did not spread too much comfort to the industrialists.

News items were breaking swiftly as 1971 began, as reflected by the pages of Louis Rothschild's *Food Chemical News*, one of the most perceptive, honest, and thorough publications in the field. Even though the almost indestructible DDT levels were causing nationwide concern, poultry and feed operators were pushing for larger tolerances. Shell and Gulf Oil rose up on their haunches to protest against possible FDA restrictions on some of their herbicide and soil fumigant products, and they were joined by Dow and Monsanto. Considerable controversy was raised when the FDA made it known that it might turn to the industry's own straw man, the Consumer Research Institute, for advice on its new plan for better nutritional labeling on food products. Robert Choate, who had critically attacked the nutritional values of cereals the year before, was most vociferous in his scorn of the FDA in going to an industry organization. "This is pure and unadulterated fraud," he said. "This is a classic example of going to the fox to ask what the chickens are doing."

Dr. Jean Mayer, the director of the White House Conference on Food, Nutrition, and Health, emphasized the importance of more sensible nutritional information on foods. Ironically, information is more detailed and specific on pet foods than on human food products. In the January, 1971, *Family Health* magazine, Jean Mayer wrote: "As we use more and more highly processed foods, it is essential that the public and health professionals alike know what is in the food we buy. For instance, when choosing a particular type of food, one should know how much of the characteristic nutrient it contains—such as chicken in chicken pie, or unsaturated fat in margarine." Dr. Mayer feels strongly that the labeling rules have not caught up with the food revolution.

Ralph Nader and his Raiders were not at all inactive in January, 1971. Among other activities, Nader pointed a finger at the FDA for not taking action on two color additives known as violet 1 and citrus red 2. You can see the violet color dye on practically all the fatty meat or poultry you buy carrying a trade-name stamp. The FDA has agreed to have the dye reexamined by the National Academy of Sciences. Citrus red 2 is the color that makes your oranges look so appealing on the grocer's racks. Nader is joined by the United Nations' World Health Organization, which has contended that the color additive has definitely been shown to have carcinogenic activity and that there are not enough data to determine a safe limit. The FDA doesn't feel there's a health hazard because the skins of oranges are usually discarded.

Speaking of the FDA's fudging on decisions about these and other color additives which are only provisionally approved, Nader said: "This should be considered a serious dereliction of duty. The situation can only serve to give the public cause to worry about chemicals that it is ingesting and cause to worry about the kind of protection it is receiving from the FDA."

Joining the parade of industry protests against anything that might stand in the way of profits was the legal action by the Toilet Goods Association which was fighting to keep the use of color additives for cosmetics secret.

The FDA's new and continuing study of the GRAS ("generally recognized as safe" food additives) list came in for a considerable number of potshots from industry. Individual companies were trying to keep the tracks clear to have plenty of elbow room to use chemical additives freely, without the FDA looking over their shoulders. Kraft, General Mills, Campbell Soups, Nestlé, and others all badgered the FDA to keep hands off their varied and multiple, and often thoughtless, decisions regarding what *they* wanted to throw into the food pot. The main thrust of the problem the FDA faced in making decisions about the safety of food additives was not whether one or two individual additives were potentially harmful—but what would be the *total* effect of all the varied additives each company wanted to use for its own product? What about the mixture of one additive with a dozen others from other foods? What was the cumulative effect? Did some additives combine to create an unsuspected lethal condition? None of the corporations brought these critical questions to the surface in their arguments. As a matter of fact, several weeks after the start of 1971, UPI reported that food industry leaders bluntly told the FDA that they reserve the right to add chemicals and other substances to foods without even advising the government.

The Food and Drug Law Institute frankly suggested that the FDA's "safe," or GRAS, list for chemical food additives was a "myth" for all practical purposes. Such a list, the institute argued, by no means included all the chemicals industry was dumping into cans and packages lining the supermarket shelves.

For the reasonably aware consumer who thought that the FDA was keeping a tight rein on the food manufacturers, this statement would come as a distinct shock. But even further shock came from the statement by Fritz, Dodge & Olcott, the company that produces many of the additives the food processors are so fond of proliferating: "It should be clear," said a spokesman for the company, "that industry has the right to make its own decisions on the status of any substance whether or not the FDA has listed it, and that it is under no obligation to request the FDA to express an opinion on unlisted materials."

Standing in line to back up this statement with similar disregard for rational control of conditions rapidly getting out of hand were the ubiquitous lobby groups like the National Canners Association, the Grocery Manufacturers of America, the Manufacturing Chemists Association, the Flavor and Extract Association, Procter & Gamble, R. T. French, and all the rest of the anti-control fraternity.

Jim Turner, former attorney with Ralph Nader's Center for the Study of Responsive Law and author of the book *The Chemical Feast*, quickly retorted to a UPI reporter: "These comments demonstrate conclusively how ineffective the food additive amendments are in practice. There may be many chemicals in our food which even the FDA is unaware of."

Meanwhile, *Food Chemical News* was reporting on the sharp questioning of another myth: the safety of iron in the diet. While the bakery corporations were plugging for adding more iron fortification (as a sales tool) to enrich bread and flour, Dr. William Crosby, chief of hematology at the New England Medical Center Hospital, joined by Dr. Margaret Ann Krikker, was opposing any such procedure. Both doctors urged that iron and iron salts should be removed from the approved GRAS list of food additives. Their reports pointed out that too much iron is destructive, that there is no way for the body to eliminate excess quantities, that it leads to a pathological condition known as hemochromatosis, that too much iron is particularly damaging to males and postmenapausal females, and that the use of iron in baby foods is acceptable only under the close surveillance of the American Academy of Pediatrics. "It is one essential nutrient mineral," said Dr. Crosby, "which cannot be regarded as safe."

The enthusiasm the mills and bakeries have shown for fortifying bread and flour derives, of course, from their bleaching to death many essential nutrients in the process of making the flour white in order to appeal to the customer. In replacing artificially the natural nutrition they have already removed, the search for emotionally toned sales gimmick additives is constant. With this sort of frenetic activity part and parcel of the whole spectrum of food production, not even the most astute body of nutritional experts can tell or predict what is happening in the overall picture.

The fair-haired pets, vitamins A and D, are sprinkled lavishly by food processors into their Space Age concoctions, though neither of them are water soluble, and both of them in excess can cause severe disorders. Their magic sales appeal on a food label is unquestioned. But their capacity for body damage is likewise unquestioned, especially when children are often given vitamin tablets to pile on top of the fortified foods. One of the fears expressed by the FDA in mid-January was that a nutrient horsepower race might be in the making that would lead to "indiscriminate fortification" of all types of foods.

Also in early 1971, Dr. Jean Lockhart, a supervising medical officer for the FDA, posed the question as to how drugs can be labeled for children when there is a critical lack of research on how these drugs might affect children. She pointed out that doctors, quite properly, are not at all enthusiastic about using children as guinea pigs to test drugs; that this in turn prevents the assembling of adequate data to know whether the drugs are safe or not; that this leads to drugs being labeled "not for children"; and that this then makes children "therapeutic orphans." She argued that the penalty for ignoring the special physiological characteristics of children as compared to adults can bring about severe adverse reactions and side effects when children are given drugs. One of these, the "gray syndrome," arises because an immature liver simply cannot handle the effects of chloramphenicol (Chloromycetin), a quixotic and deadly antibiotic under any circumstances.

Many drugs, she attested, are less toxic than others as far as infants are concerned. Among the more toxic are phenobarbital, acetylsalicylic acid (aspirin), meprobamate, and chlorpromazine. Ordinary adult ferrous sulfate (iron) tablets are even more toxic. Even oxygen can be highly toxic to the young infant. Less toxic to the young are dextroamphetamine, digitalis, codeine, and others. Interesting in her comments is that children are now discovered to develop diseases formerly thought to occur only in adults, such as psychoneurosis, peptic ulcers, and gout. The danger here is that drug treatments for these "adult" diseases have practically never been tested for children. Her contention was that the reluctance to test drugs on children can cause far more ultimate harm than otherwise.

As January, 1971, drew to a close, one of the more blatant

statements of industrial arrogance came to the limelight regarding the actions of the Food and Drug Administration when a condition of "imminent hazard" is declared, as for instance, when a shipment of an external antiseptic might be found to be chemically decomposed, as happened with thousands of bottles of Merck, Sharp & Dohme's Cresatin over a period of months. This is obviously an imminent hazard, and in such cases the FDA requests the company to make a "voluntary" recall. (If the company doesn't go along with the request, the FDA will flood the country with publicity. And even if the recall is made, it is necessary for the FDA to publicize the problem to avoid further use of the product.)

If there is anything that all corporations hate it is this type of publicity. They often attempt to block it, even if it is most urgent for the consuming public to know.

Bucking this important FDA tool for safeguarding the consumer through publicity, General Foods approached the FDA to say in silken tones: ". . . it may not be either wise or useful for the FDA to publicize these imminent hazard situations broadly in every instance," adding that publicity like this "can in fact create undue public hysteria." Then, in its calm, dignified, pinstripe attitude, the request continued by suggesting that a *manufacturer* "can serve a useful purpose in working out with the FDA the appropriate form and extent of publicity." In other words, let us couch the entire imminent hazard situation in melodious and euphemistic tones, limit the circulation of the publicity, and commend the consumer who fails to appreciate the significance of a warning to his own content.

Controversy and question marks ranged over a wide variety of things that brought concern to the consumer, as 1971 moved from days to weeks to months. The Federal Trade Commission, sister organization to the FDA, found itself clamping down on unwarranted nutritional claims by the Carnation Instant Breakfast people. FDA inspectors were prodded to review the screening of the National Canners Association of the tuna packed in this country. One FDA chemist in the New York laboratories was seen leaning against the coffee machine in the corridor outside his lab, smoking a cigarette. He plaintively said to his companion: "If I smell one more tuna fish, I'm going to lose my cookies."

But it was the next dozen weeks or so that ushered in the kind of crisis that brings nightmares to the FDA, the manufacturer, and the general public alike.

3

Vampire Blood, and the Hex of Hexachlorophene and Other Stories

FEBRUARY, 1971, began peacefully enough.

A staff FDA public relations man was heard mumbling in the corridor about something that sounded like "vampire blood."

The strange part was that was exactly what he *was* saying. He had just ripped out of his typewriter a press release marked PUBLIC WARNING, a story regarding over 1,000,000 1-ounce plastic tubes on the market handsomely mounted on display cartons and brightly labeled VAMPIRE BLOOD. This pleasant little plaything for the kiddy market was manufactured by a company called Nutrilite Products, Inc., and distributed by an outfit with the unlikely name of Imagineering, Inc. These plastic tubes were sold in novelty stores and other retail outfits with the sole purpose of providing a product that would simulate human blood.

What stirred the interest of the FDA inspectors was that this Dracula-like product was discovered to be especially dangerous if it came in contact with any kind of skin abrasion, particularly around the eyes or mouth. The cheerful byproduct of this educational toy came to the FDA's attention through the Virginia Department of Health, which had discovered that Vampire Blood was generally riddled with a pathogenic bacterium known as *Pseudomonas seruginosa*. The product was immediately recalled from the consumer level on up, but not until a considerable handful of innocent young monsters discovered that vampires weren't quite as much fun as they used to be.

The usual recalls of other products were, of course, continuing, as they always did. Nearly 700 cartons of a ceramic dishware set from Italy were recalled when it was discovered that any kind of acid in foods would leach out a generous supply of lead. Several California potteries faced the same fate with their leachable lead earthenware from Mexico and elsewhere. Armour Pharmaceutical was called on the carpet for misbranding its Coricotropin Injection, as well as Burroughs Wellcome for its Cortisporin Optic drops, found to be subpotent. Swordfish had its saddest time, with multiple recalls the rule of the day.

Kraft cheese was forced to recall hundreds of cases of its Deluxe Sliced American Cheese, its Tubby Ribbon Cheese, and its Loaf American products because of pesticide contamination. Safeway stores met the same fate with some of its Lucerne Party Dip Bacon and Horseradish in 8-ounce containers found to contain rodent contamination.

As if the engulfing tide of mercury in the environment weren't bad enough, the Associated Press had uncovered several months before that mercury was being used as a preservative in several types of cosmetics. This and other concerns about hair dyes, aerosol hair sprays, bubble baths, and shampoos were sparking a considerable amount of laboratory activity.

Industry is worried about the new wave of consumerism. The Machiavellian and clumsy attempts by General Motors to smear Ralph Nader several years ago (American Home Products tried to do the same thing to a Congressional committee investigator) was an example of the grotesque acrobatics the so-called respectable corporations of the country will engage in, merely because an articulate spokesman takes action to protect the consumer from practices that should have been self-regulated years before. It would be charitable to say that much of this attitude of industry comes from corporate blindness, and much of it does. But other evidence points to outright venality, and this cannot be denied by any collection of industry's suave public relations polemics.

Speaking to a National Canners Association meeting in early 1971, the chief legal counsel of that organization shot charges at the press and radio for aiding and abetting the "vigor of consumerism"—as if consumers had little or no right to demand protection from industry abuses. He went on to grouse about Congressional, agency, and court action and voiced surprise that the "acrimonious agitation and critical publicity is taking hold with a surprising number of consumers"—as if that were an undesirable trait on the part of the guinea pigs which had grown from 100,000,000 to 200,000,000 in less than half a century.

The Canners Association spokesman fretted about the possible establishment of a consumer protection agency, called Congressional investigations into the new hazards in food, drugs, and cosmetics "constant harassments," and lashed out at Ralph Nader, Jim Turner, and Robert Choate.

Dr. Jean Mayer, the expert who was responsible for guiding the White House Conference on Nutrition, took note of industry's promotion practices when he said that the majority of advertisements of the food industry directed its attention to "highly processed snack foods and such things as candy, soft drinks, and alcoholic beverages, which can only be consumed at the expense of primary foods."

But all this was heat lightning compared to two loud thunder claps that struck the FDA offices, beginning in February.

For nearly two decades, hexachlorophene has been a fair-haired antiseptic that seemingly could cause no harm. Hospitals and doctors have used it lavishly in the form of the liquid soap pHisoHex. Empires have literally been built on hexachlorophene in the form of Dial soap, other soaps, feminine hygiene sprays, mouthwashes, toothpastes, shampoos, Breck and other hair dressings, and other handy items for household and personal use. Cosmetics are loaded with it, although we don't know which and how much, because the cosmetic companies escape the responsibility of having to label the contents with ingredients, as other FDA-regulated materials do.

The dangers of the chemical began unfolding slowly, almost imperceptibly. Hexachlorophene is a close chemical relative to the deadly herbicides 2,4,5-T and 2,4-D, which have ravaged the foliage of Vietnam. It is actually made from the same material. An incredibly weak warning by the FDA was issued in spring, 1971. Its full impact was not to be felt until late in the year. A new, stronger warning was issued in December—but not until Ralph Nader had blasted the situation wide open, chafing the FDA for catering to the multibillion-dollar industry using the dangerous chemical without regard to its dangers.

One of the more colorful, articulate, and perceptive spokesmen for the toilet goods industries is Amelia Bassin, an independent consultant who is one of the few sensitive enough to prod the sluggish members of the clan into some kind of enlightened self-greed, at least. Speaking to a New York convention, the ex-vice-president of Fabergé told a group of food and drug officials that cosmetic manufacturers should set up their own policing unit, very much on the order of the Underwriters Lab. Its job would be to pretest and approve products coming onto the market. It would, she felt, be the only way to avoid inevitable government regulation. If the cause she was supporting was more than debatable (history has proved that industry's self-regulation is far more of a farce than a fact), her rhetoric was charming and persuasive.

Speaking of the inevitable crackdown on the loose and liberal regulations the cosmetic industry enjoyed at least for the moment, she said: "I'll bet the FDA is about to open something, and I suspect it's not just a little old can of worms. It's probably a small, exquisitely-packaged, ground-glass-stoppered, sparkling crystal 24-carat gold-line, satin-bedded travel-sized highly concentrated and extremely explosive, stunningly labeled *court action.* Why can't industry and the government get together and come up with a workable solution short of you-know-what? Why can't we have a computerized rating system to test and evaluate and report? Why can't somebody do a simple little thing like define hypo-al-lergenic?"

Referring to the sluggish initiative of the Toilet Goods As-sociation, she urged them to organize their own micro-FDA within the industry but didn't feel too optimistic about it. "I've become a member of the Toilet Goods Association re-cently, hoping at least to find out something if not to help, but so far all I've heard from them is 'send money.' "

Driving hard at a critical point as far as the consumer is concerned, she pointed out that consumers couldn't care less about what was in lipstick or face cream or deodorant sprays. "But they want the government and the manufacturers to care. If industry had its wits on, it would go right ahead and comply like mad. It would print the ingredients right there on the package—everybody knows consumers are barely able to pronounce 'aluminum chlorohydrate,' " she said.

Then she continued: "Most consumers—certainly the un-liberated ones—would like merely to feel confident that *any* cosmetic they buy is safe, without having to make judgments for which they are inadequately qualified. They want to feel confident that each and every cosmetic they buy is pure and safe and fresh as advertised. All those other goodies such as fun and fashion and instant sex appeal are so much icing on the cake." She noted that all the vivid claims of cosmetic ad-vertising were drawing a considerable amount of attention from agencies like the FDA and the Federal Trade Commis-sion.

And she was right. Well aware that the next big time bomb might be likely to lie in either the cosmetic or thera-peutic device industry, the government agencies were am-plifying their scrutiny of everything from shampoos to hair dyes. If the hexachlorophene story could be a basic example, they would be moving slowly, but at least inexorably.

Regarding the relatively new idea of vaginal spray deodor-ants, but ignoring the potential and very real dangers of hex-achlorophene and other ingredients in them, Miss Bassin said: "The cosmetic industry has just recently made the per-fectly astounding discovery that women have an extra orifice, and is making much hay thereby. Such current delicacies as flavored douches and feminine deodorant sprays prove that funny things do happen on the way to the orifice."

But the guts of her speech lay in one simple sentence, a sentence so true that it captured in a few words the essence of the entire problem of foods, drugs, cosmetics, toilet goods, mechanical health devices, hazardous substances, toys, and pesticide and herbicide contamination as far as the consumer is concerned. The cosmetic industry, she said, "is completely incapable of making an innovative move without the pressure of a 10-alarm fire. Beauty biz is characterized by a broad yellow stripe running down its collective back."

James Merritt, president of the Toilet Goods Association, which was just then in the process of changing its name to the Cosmetic, Toiletry, and Fragrance Association, had no comment.

While the cosmetic business was having its fears and worries, the routine FDA recalls were moving along *ad nauseam*. Principal villains of new lists were continued mercury in swordfish, misbranded and subpotent drugs, more lead in pottery, pesticide contamination in a wide spectrum of foods, and hazardous toys. Kraft was still having trouble with its American cheese, Dow Chemical with its Intromycin antibiotic product.

Fifty thousand cases of Hawaiian Punch had to be recalled when its label declared, deadpan and serious: "Low calorie; No cyclamates; contains water—sodium cyclamate."

The Pepsi-Cola Company also had bad luck. Nearly 30,000 cases of Pepsi, Teem, Mason's Root Beer, Hi-Q Orange Soda, and the Dr. Pepper it bottled under special license were whisked off the market when consumers began discovering that the taste of machine oil did not exactly enhance the flavor. A breakdown of plant machinery provided the added and unwanted bonus to the bottles.

Concern about prescription drugs was rising, not only about a plethora of new drugs that were being slipped onto the market without prior FDA approval, as required by law, but by the continuance of the now-habitual practice on the part of the "ethical" drug companies to promote the effectiveness of drugs that weren't effective and the failure of the drug companies to warn of serious, even lethal, side effects and adverse reactions in their splashy ads directed at physicians in the elegant medical journals.

Sam D. Fine, Associate Commissioner for Compliance of the FDA, laid down a smarting dictum to the pharmaceutical companies in an official notice in the *Federal Register* in mid-February.

"The Food and Drug Administration," he wrote, "is seriously concerned about the continued introduction into the market of new products without submission and approval through the new drug procedure of the Federal Food, Drug, and Cosmetic Act. This appears to result from a misunderstanding of the new drug requirements or from a deliberate effort to avoid the new drug procedure."

He must have been being charitable about the "misunderstanding" idea, because no drug manufacturer could possibly misunderstand the specific regulation that all new Rx drugs, and even old drugs with suggested new uses, must receive advance approval before being marketed. Continuing with his warning, he stated: "Should a manufacturer or distributor undertake to decide unilaterally that any such product does not require new-drug approval, he must recognize that he risks criminal and civil regulatory action."

Fifteen different medical journal ads were forced to be canceled by the FDA for extravagant or incomplete information about drugs during the first two months of 1971. Two major drug firms were required to run ads to correct misleading ads they had run previously during that time. Two other leading firms were on the brink of legal action because of their bad track record in attempting to mislead doctors about the use of their Rx remedies.

A delightful, bitter, and telling segment by Nicholas Von Hoffman, columnist and commentator, on NET's television show *The Great American Dream Machine* on ads in the medical journals told the story eloquently. In a beautifully produced sequence, a montage of medical journal ads flowed by the camera, accompanied by lilting music, as Von Hoffman's rasping and articulate voice pointed out a few anomalies.

One ad floated by the camera showing a sexy woman framed by the headline: MAYBE SHE WON'T. As it did, Von Hoffman said:

"Maybe she won't. Won't what? Put her clothes on? Get out of her bag? Get into her bag? Maybe she won't. But if she does get an infective dermatitis, Fluinid N, neomycin sulphate, fluocinolone acetonide can break the infection cycle.

"We're used to the patent medicine man's pitch," Von Hoffman continued in his commentary. " 'See, Dad, we did it. Only one cavity.' Or: 'Mama Mia, Alka Seltzer, if we've eaten too many speecy, spicy meatballs.' Or there's the little Hindu if we can't sleep, sleep, sleep. We laymen swallow the patent medicine ads. But we assume that the doctor's choice of drugs for us is based on straight, clinical facts."

Von Hoffman then went on to display two medical magazines, edited for the exclusive doctor audience. Referring to an appropriate illustration as another ad floated by the camera, still with lilting music, Von Hoffman said: "Romance. Cut short by back pain? Medicine will bring them together. Lyricism." Then he read part of the advertising copy—and remember, now, this is advice for a serious prescription drug for an ill patient:

"It was a shame about Harry Van Leer.
His vacation was ruined by diarrhea
Got tenesmus and spasm
At Ausable Chasm
Send Donnagel with him this year."

Another ad floated by. Attractive young couple. Von Hoffman continued, voice over the music: "Attractive. A sporty family can sell anything. Even penicillin. But nothing, nothing, Baby, sells like sex."

Another ad with a sexy woman. The narration continued: "What does she make you think of? Soft breezes, South Sea islands, right? You're wrong. It's Terramycin, the broad spectrum antibiotic."

More ads floated by the camera. A headline for an embracing couple: WILL ANGINA COME BETWEEN THEM TONIGHT? Another ad from a leading pharmaceutical house, as all of these were. It showed an appropriate illustration for the headline: HE FELL OFF HIS HORSE IN AN ANTIHISTAMINE DAZE. Another montage, music up and under. Another beautiful girl in the medical ad to catch the unsuspecting doctor's eye. Again Von Hoffman, saying: "And she—doesn't she mean a vioform hydrocortisone to you? And the less sexy ladies, the compassionate pitch. Sedate some. Give them antidepressants. Give them tranquilizers. Don't settle for half measures. Zap 'em!"

Von Hoffman pointed out that these ads were not as amusing as they seemed. Physicians claimed they weren't swayed by this sort of drivel. But why, then, did the ethical drug houses spend half a billion dollars a year on this type of advertising? With the evidence suggesting massive overprescription to patients, it was little wonder that 10 percent of hospital admissions were for adverse drug reactions.

"Expert testimony before a Senate subcommittee," Von Hoffman told the *American Dream Machine* audience, "estimates that more than one-half the money spent on prescriptions is wasted. It's suspected that the number of deaths from prescription drugs surpasses death from heroin, or from diseases like nephritis or cancer of the breast. The estimate is that at least 29,000 people died from prescribed drugs last year.

"So these ads aren't funny," he went on. "They're symptomatic of an industry that can't control itself. It's like a manic, metastasizing cell, an organism that uses advertising to join mass production, profit-seeking and medicine in a dangerously inappropriate fashion."

At the conclusion of the segment, an announcer voice-over stated: "The preceding ads included additional medical information."

The staff at NET argued long and loudly about inserting this phrase on the basis that it was somewhat of an apology when no apology of the sort was necessary. NET's legal department was apprehensive, and caution prevailed.

Just how inadequate a major blue-chip drug company can be in its own quality control of production began showing up in deadly earnest not too long after NET had aired its witty jabs at the entire industry.

The roots of the story go back to 1964. Abbott Laboratories, the pharmaceutical house that had the questionable honor of being the largest supplier of cyclamates and the one that fought hardest against the ultimate ban on that product for use in either regular or diet foods, is the focus of the story. Its track record over the years might be considered a little less than inspiring.

In the mid-sixties, one of Abbott's medical customers was preparing a bottle of fluid for intravenous injection for a seriously ill patient. The bottle was labeled "5% Dextrose in Water." Two of the basic intravenous injection fluids are dextrose, as the one labeled here, or saline solution, another name for common salt, or sodium chloride, solutions. Both are critically important and often mean a matter of life or death. The scene where these fluids are administered is familiar: the bottle clamped on a metal stand beside the patient's hospital bed; the long rubber tube running down to the arm, where it disappears under adhesive tape covering the needle entering the vein.

In this case, it was discovered that far from containing dextrose, the bottle contained sodium chloride. It was a fortunate discovery. Over 300 bottles of saline solution were masquerading as dextrose solution, potentially setting up a manifold medical disaster. The roots of the cause lay in the labeling machine: 500 wrong labels were fed into it through what Abbott called "human error." Over 11,000 bottles had to be recalled to discover those that were mislabeled.

On the heels of this potential disaster, 500 more Abbott intravenous bottles had the wrong label but the right embossing identification on the bottle caps. Thirty-three more lots were recalled and destroyed, but this was only the beginning. As more label-and-bottle-cap mix-ups turned up, as frantic telegrams went out to doctors and hospitals, other lots were found to have mold in them.

When the FDA asked Abbott to recall the latter, Abbott got testy. It tried to blame the hospitals for damaging the bottles. FDA investigators didn't quite see it the same way, because there was no evidence of damage. But since the lot was rather aged—four years old—the FDA felt it didn't have a strong enough case to prosecute. In the meantime, Abbott was not exactly profiting from the experience. The cost of warning telegrams is alleged to have run to more than $750,000.

But as the Western Union wires were cooling down, another problem literally seeped into the picture. Abbott had changed the plastic liners on its screw-top caps from Gilsonite to Mylar. Since Abbott supplies nearly half of the entire intravenous fluid market, this was a major change. Other companies use rubber stoppers, which seemed entirely satisfactory.

Even in high school biology classes, the importance of true sterilization when required is hammered into the students' heads with passionate regularity. In the same high school labs, the importance of checking and rechecking for possible shortcomings in sterilization is emphasized repeatedly, and if conditions fail to provide this, they must be corrected.

It is hard to find the reason why Abbott, with its sophisticated labs and technicians, could not discern what was about to happen next. It took the FDA to discover that there was a cap leakage problem with the new cap liners. It involved the new Mylar plastic, which wasn't working as well as the old one.

A cap leakage in a sterile intravenous solution is a potential catastrophe. Bacteria swarm to the leakage point, even though the bottle is originally sterile. They lurk in the crevices of the cap, wait for the fluid to pour out into the tube, join it for a tumbling ride down the tube and directly into the vein. Results: septicemia, or blood poisoning, often of such severity that antibiotics are useless in fighting it. In addition to the systemic blood poisoning, phlebitis spreads dramatically at the point where the needle goes into the vein.

Another series of recalls followed—310 lots between October, 1964, and April, 1965. Finally, Abbott persuaded its manufacturer to go back to making Gilsonite cap liners. With this step, there was a brief breathing period.

But it did not last long. This time it was hairline cracks in the necks of the glass bottles. The FDA didn't discover the problem until 1969. Abbott had been hearing about it, loud and clear, from its customers for some eight months before this. Something was going wrong with the annealing of the glass in the neck of the bottles. The result: the same as with the plastic liners. More contamination, more colonies of bacteria to spoil the sterilization, more threats to the thousands of patients who lay sick and dependent in hospital beds.

And more recalls, all through 1969. The problem lay not only in the defective glass bottles but with the inspection and quality-control processes that could spot the trouble. Abbott finally spent several hundred thousand dollars to beef up its inspection and quality-control processes, but just why they were so sluggish in getting around to it has never been publicly explained. And just why even this frenzied step turned out to be meaningless will remain one of the greater mysteries of the chemical age.

But the FDA failed to prosecute in 1969. They figured there wasn't sufficient evidence to pin Abbott on criminal action or to refer the case to the Department of Justice. Besides, Abbott had "assured" them that they had fully corrected the causes of the difficulties and that patients could now lie back in their hospital beds to gaze up at the Abbott label, suffused with confidence that the great pharmaceutical company's self-regulation would see them through the night.

Pharmaceutical companies have assured many people of many things: of their spurious need for astronomical profits at the expense of a consumer who often must use the product or die*; of their dedication to research work, which often consists of changing or adding a useless atom in a molecule in

* This is called "the glass of water in the Sahara" economic philosophy by many economists. When you are desperate for a prescription, you don't argue about money.

order to get around a patent or obtain a new one; of their innocence in conspiring to keep prices high for critically needed drugs—for instance, as was brought out during the Kefauver hearings, Tetracycline cost the literally helpless consumer 50 cents a pill when it actually cost Bristol-Myers 1.7 cents to make.

But Abbott's assurance that all was well when the FDA dropped its charges in 1969 was not swallowed as readily by Washington reporter Morton Mintz as it was by the FDA. Mintz is a tough journalist who knows how to dig and how to confront, and he did both in this case.

In the fall of 1970, Mintz wrote the general counsel of the FDA a letter asking what had happened to the planned criminal charges against Abbott. He had learned of a secret citation hearing into the matter by the FDA and asked for the transcript of this and other records, which are considered by many to be available under what is called the Freedom of Information Act regarding public records.

Mintz heard nothing from the FDA counsel's office until some four months later. General Counsel W. W. Goodrich pleaded that the transcript Mintz had requested contained secret commercial information that could not be released. It was exempt from the Freedom of Information Act, Goodrich added.

At almost exactly the same time that the FDA counsel was writing this reply, a medical paper in the prestigious *New England Journal of Medicine*, the February 4, 1971, issue, detailed the story of septicemia, or blood poisoning, arising from a *new* wave of patients receiving Abbott's intravenous fluids. And the facts showed that this had nothing to do with the 1969 outbreak. In other words, the merry-go-round was starting all over again, barely a year after the FDA had so graciously dropped its criminal charges against Abbott.

The news of the new trouble had begun leaking in December. No less than five patients, all of them in a coronary intensive care unit at the University of Virginia Medical Hospital, were riddled with septicemia within the span of a few days. Tests showed that two kinds of bacilli were guilty: erwinia and enterobacter cloacae, both extremely rare among blood poisoning cases. It did not take long to trace the source of the deadly bacilli: Abbott intravenous fluids.

The shockers began coming in in January, 1971: Henry Ford Hospital in Detroit counted eight deaths over the previous three-month period, along with forty-five other cases of blood poisoning traced to the Abbott fluids. In Denver, St. Anthony's Hospital reported twenty-four cases and one death. As the weeks went on through January and February, the reports mounted.

Atlanta's Center for Disease Control, part of the U.S. Public Health Service, did the detective work and the lab work, but Dr. Dennis Maki and microbiologist Donald Mackel told a *Newsweek* reporter that they were "extremely puzzled" about how the bacilli raided the Abbott bottles. Bottles taken off the shelf had proved negative, as had the tubing, needles, and surfaces of the bottle. They also said they checked hand lotions and soaps used throughout the hospital for bacteria but found none. A previous epidemic had stemmed from this cause.

It took several weeks before they even thought of checking the new-style screw-on cap, the same location that had started all the trouble back in the mid-1960's. What is most incredible is why Maki and Mackel didn't know about the long history of the tragicomedy Abbott had been playing with its bottle caps and bottle necks. Why did it take them so many weeks to check this area? Or, as *Newsweek* put it:

> Maki suddenly realized that the one part of the IV [intravenous] equipment that had not yet been checked for bacteria were the tops of the fluid bottles. . . . In short order, Maki and the microbiologist Donald Mackel found the guilty germs lurking between the liner and the disk in about half of the lots of the solution they tested. If the bottle was shaken or the top banged loose for easier removal, they also found, the solution washed over the liner and became contaminated.

Suddenly? In short order? Weeks, even months, had gone

by before this was discerned, yet the history was glaring at them—or was it?—in the files of the FDA.

Even then, the warnings did not go out until March 13, 1971, when the head of the Center for Disease Control and FDA's Commissioner Charles Edwards issued a joint release stating that Abbott Laboratories was "working to correct the problem."

Working to correct the problem? They had been doing that since the 1960's. Abbott had escaped criminal prosecution in a secret hearing at the FDA. They were back again at the same old stand, the largest supplier of IV fluids in the country, the once-proud king of the cyclamates.

But even with the March 13, 1971, warning, the bottles were not recalled. The joint release simply urged health authorities to open the containers at the time of use only. It took until March 16, 1971, for the detailed release of information for hospitals to go out over the TWX (teletype) wires to the local FDA offices. Packed with more technical information, it began:

> . . . BACTEREMIAS ATTRIBUTED TO INTRAVENOUS FLUID THERAPY BETWEEN OCTOBER AND MARCH 1, 1971; EIGHT UNITED STATES HOSPITALS IN SEVEN STATES EXPERIENCE 150 BACTEREMIAS CAUSED BY ENTEROBACTER CLOACAE OR GRAM NEGATIVE ORGANISMS OF THE ERWINIA GROUP. THERE WERE NINE DEATHS, ALL OF THEM ASSOCIATED WITH INTRAVENOUS (IV) FLUID THERAPY . . . ALL EIGHT HOSPITALS UTILIZE FLUID AND SYSTEMS MANUFACTURED BY ABBOTT LABORATORIES, WHICH PRODUCES APPROXIMATELY 45 PER CENT OF ALL IV FLUIDS SOLD WITHIN THE UNITED STATES . . . THESE SEPTICEMIAS WERE CONSISTENTLY CHARACTERIZED BY INTERMITTENT HIGH FEVER, ALTHOUGH SHOCK WAS INFREQUENT . . . ANTI-MICROBIALS [ANTIBIOTICS] HAVE FREQUENTLY BEEN WITHOUT APPARENT EFFECT ON THE COURSE OF THE INFECTION. . . .

But still there was no real FDA action. There were important considerations here the FDA did have to face. Since Abbott, in spite of its inglorious record, still supplied over 45 percent of the market, where would the replacement fluids come from? Did the minority companies have enough bottles on hand to fill the gap? Would a patient die because of a lack of the vital fluid? If there were other supplies in warehouses, could they reach a hospital in time to prevent this?

By March 19, 1971, Ralph Nader got hold of the story through a doctor who had learned that one New York hospital had dozens more cases of blood poisoning than the government reports showed—and that the mild precautions suggested by the FDA were literally worthless. Patients were coming down like flies with the infection. (Much later, it was learned that the precautions suggested by Commissioner Edwards were indeed worthless. One twist of the cap, and the bacteria were loosed by the millions.)

Nader's letter to Edwards was sent March 21. He said that it was a form of malpractice to wait until a patient develops evidence of blood infection and that the recommendation was a "cowardly repudiation of the ethics of preventive medicine." A few days later, Nader went on the air on a TV news program. Edwards fumbled badly in trying to field Nader's charges.

But nowhere in the news did the long history of Abbott's delinquencies throughout the 1960's come to the foreground. Nor was there any explanation of Edwards' statement that he didn't know about the problem until March 11 or that the FDA survey and search for alternate supplies was not made until March 19. On this date it was discovered that the bulk of Abbott intravenous fluids could be replaced by other pharmaceutical companies.

It took until March 22, 1971—the day after Nader's TV appearance—for the FDA to issue a release on the recommendation of the Center for Disease Control that "hospitals and other health care facilities not use Abbott Laboratories intravenous infusion products unless absolutely necessary."

The evidence had grown now to 350 cases of blood poisoning in twenty-one hospitals, and it was still growing. Some experts believe there were thousands of unreported cases, including many more deaths. Commissioner Edwards was almost apologetic in his statement recommending against the use of the Abbott fluids. "On the basis of these recommendations, the FDA is compelled to recommend that the Abbott product not be used at this time," he said. But the next statement in the release is most puzzling in the light of the historical seven-year battle between the FDA and Abbott. "Abbott fully expects to solve its problem and will be allowed to reenter the market as soon as it does so."

Abbott had been "fully expecting to solve its problem" since 1964. How long would it take for a clout to mean something? One FDA executive muttered, half under his breath, "Those Abbott people are such *bastards.*"

Finally, in the first week in April, the FDA garnered up enough courage to recall the Abbott products. The Army hospitals had already done this, two weeks before, on March 16, by medical directive.

It would be good to report that this is the end of a long, sad story of dire consumer hazard, a symbol, of course, of what continues to go on in many other consumer areas. But it isn't.

As hospitals all over the country pleaded with other suppliers to help them replace the deadly Abbott bottles, the picture darkened a little.

One hospital superintendent frantically phoned a different pharmaceutical house, since his intravenous supply was shrinking to zero. "We're really on a spot," he told the detail man. "I've got to have at least five or six dozen IV bottles of various solutions here by six o'clock tonight, or I don't know what's going to happen to the patients. I can't use the Abbott stuff, obviously. Could you possibly help me out?"

"Absolutely," came the cheery voice of the detail man. "Don't worry about it at all."

The superintendent was stunned and grateful that he could get this emergency help. "You *can?*" he asked incredulously.

"No problem at all," said the detail man. "I'll just get the order down on the pad and have the stuff up there by mid-afternoon."

"I can't thank you enough," said the superintendent.

"Only one minor thing and we can clear that up in no time," the detail man added.

"What's that?" asked the superintendent.

"All we need is a three-year, firm contract," was the reply. "As soon as you sign it, the shipment is yours."

Waiting in the wings while all this was going on was an investigation by the Department of Justice that had nothing to do with intravenous fluids but plenty to do with Abbott. One of Abbott's new products was a serum called Aus-Tect. Its use was designed to determine whether donated blood contained any of the virus that causes serum hepatitis. Abbott had begun shipping the serum interstate without trifling with the legal necessity of getting its new drug application approved by the FDA. In addition, it failed to label the drug so that the user would know that it was only 35 percent effective. Such inconvenience to the user could have a hefty impact when the life or death of a patient might depend on knowing for certain if the blood was safe to use.

In early May, the ax fell, and Abbott was charged with a thirty-six-count criminal charge. Later the serum was eventually licensed under proper labeling.

Meanwhile, Abbott continues persuading physicians to prescribe its drug Nembutal. A patient can get the generic equivalent form of it as pentobarbital at a fraction of the cost. It also joins with Lilly to corner the market on an antibiotic known as erythromycin stearate. Both brands sell for the strangely identical price of $21.99 for 100 of the 250-mg. tablets.

While the Abbott and the hexachlorophene stories hugged the limelight, there was still enough left over on the early spring scene to chill the blood of any well-meaning consumer.

On March 14, a Maryland man entered a restaurant in District Heights, Maryland, just outside of Washington. With his meal, he was served some garlic-flavored toast sprinkled liberally with a powder from a Spice of Life meat tenderizer container. An unknown quantity of this condiment had been sold between March, 1969, and October, 1970, to restaurants and bars, along with its sister product for consumers, Country Tavern Meat Tenderizer. Distribution covered seven states: Virginia, Minnesota, New Jersey, Ohio, New York, Michigan, and Kansas, and the product was manufactured by Mutual Spice Company of North Bergen, New Jersey, a subsidiary of Hygrade Foods.

Within hours, the man was dead. Several containers of the product had been filled with 100-percent sodium nitrite, a deadly chemical that was packed in the Spice of Life jar instead of the tenderizer. (Sodium nitrite is also the chemical food processors like to pile on processed meats to make them look better. It is sometimes referred to as "meat lipstick." The margin between safe and unsafe use is extremely narrow.)

What made the case so particularly tragic was that a public warning notice had gone out the previous November reporting that the labeling mix-up had caused the error. Although the product was recalled, there may still be some lurking in a restaurant or home cupboard, a potential threat that develops when recalls are not fully carried out.

But there were more overtones as far as the FDA was concerned. The tragedy happened on March 15. The agency learned of this on March 15. An urgent public notice did not go out to the public until March 19. Further, the earlier FDA recall obviously was a failure, or the product would not still have been on the shelves of the restaurant.

Of more than particular interest to the office of Senator Gaylord Nelson was the news that arrived in February, 1971, that Sweden and Italy had placed a firm ban on all U.S. meats from cattle fed on stilbestrol, a synthetic compound with properties of the female sex hormone. As the Code of Federal Regulations states, stilbestrol—also known as either DES or diethylstilbestrol—is "capable of producing and has produced cancer in animals and this drug may be expected to produce, excite or stimulate the growth of certain cancers in human beings."

Stilbestrol is dumped liberally into cattle feeds to fatten

them up faster for meat industry profits. The main catch is
that most of the extra weight produced by this charming carcinogenic compound is water—in other words, a way of producing more weight and less meat per pound for the consumer.

A clause known as the Delaney clause—named after the
Senator who pushed through the vital 1958 Food Additives
Amendment—clearly provides in the Food, Drug, and Cosmetic Act of that year that *no* food additive could be approved by the FDA for any human use if the additive has
been shown to induce cancer when ingested by man or animal.

But the Kefauver-Harris drug amendments of 1962 somehow let slip an exemption from the Delaney clause to permit
drugs or chemicals to be added to animal feeds. This was
qualified to the extent that they must not produce any discernible harm to the animal and there must be no residues
left in the meat after it reached the consumer.

In other words, in the United States—but *not* Italy or Sweden—it is perfectly all right to pack an animal up with a
cancer-producing drug so that there will be more water,
more weight, and more profits to the meat packers.

The policing of whether there are any harmful residues of
stilbestrol is entirely up to the cattle raisers. They were *supposed* to stop feeding it to the animals forty-eight hours before
the animal is slaughtered. The U.S Department of Agriculture is lucky if it gets around to inspecting between 500 and
600 animals for residues of stilbestrol of all the livestock
slaughtered each year. This arrangement leaves considerable
leeway for tons of cattle to walk on the hoof into the slaughter house riddled with stilbestrol, especially when the price is
right.

Although it is hard to see why the American consumer
shouldn't get the same protection that the Swedish or Italian
consumer gets from his government, the story isn't over yet.

The FDA, with gracious condescension to a subsidiary of
Eli Lilly and Company,* a member of the pharmaceutical

* Lilly frequently places full-page ads in national magazines that read, "We've been
making medicines for years as though our lives depended on it."

pack that has fought practically all the drug legislation designed to protect the consumer, decided in September, 1970, to permit this company to *double* the dose of the drug in animal feeding. The same liberalization applies to the pellets they implant in the ears of cattle and sheep. Lilly claimed its drug left no residue in the meat *if* not fed for the previous forty-eight hours, in spite of a larger dose.

Meanwhile, FDA Commissioner Edwards talked about the situation in February, 1971. He was responding to the announcement of the American National Cattlemen's Association, which had set up a so-called self-certification program asking "every cattle feeder in the country to certify in writing that their cattle have not been fed DES [stilbestrol] for at least 48 hours prior to slaughter."

For a man of obvious intelligence and knowledge, Commissioner Edwards seemed totally unaware of the gruesome past history of industry's pseudo-self-discipline gestures. "Your indication of willingness to embark on this program will go a long way in assuring the consuming public that red meat products are wholesome and free of residues," he told the cattlemen.

It is imperative to ask how Edwards could be lured into making a statement like that, in view of the multitudinous price-fixing and market-rigging cases of the meat packers, in view of the obstructionism characterizing every major trade and industrial association in the food, drug, and cosmetic fields, to say nothing of the National Association of Manufacturers or the U.S. Chamber of Commerce. It cannot be charged off to naïveté, because Edwards is not a naïve man. And in the face of the Swedish, Italian, and threatened Common Market bans on U.S. meats, how could he support *increasing* the stilbestrol allowance for the Eli Lilly company?

His further comment is even more puzzling.

"I feel it is important to emphasize," he continued, "that whenever we document the fact that residues are present in edible parts of a slaughtered animal we will take appropriate action. I feel also that vigorous enforcement on the part of the FDA will enhance the possibility of success to your proposed program."

But how could the FDA ever document a significant number of cases where residues were left, when even the Department of Agriculture, with some 30,000 inspectors, could only check for stilbestrol on a few hundred animals a year out of some 112,000,000 cattle on the hoof?—and when Edwards himself later stated bluntly that we have *no* good control method for detecting DES residues in meat?

And vigorous FDA enforcement? The way it went with Abbott? With hexachlorophene? With cyclamates? And with myriad other drugs and food additives in the past? Perhaps the Italians and the Swedes are wiser than our own authorities. Even Edwards' own misgivings about the thin FDA budget and staff seemed to be missing from this roseate speech to the cattlemen.

But the story about stilbestrol is far from over. Later, a month or so after Edwards' glowing speech in February, 1971, to the cattlemen, three Harvard doctors announced the ominous discovery that a strange and unusual form of cancer had stricken eight young women, beginning in 1966. Their previous records showed that this form of cancer, involving prolonged vaginal bleeding, had *never* been diagnosed in young women before.

Things began falling into place when it was discovered that the *mothers* of seven out of eight of these young women (their ages ranged from twelve to twenty-two) had been given stilbestrol in very large doses during the first three months of pregnancy to avoid miscarriage. Study of a control group of girls whose mothers had not taken the drug during pregnancy showed that no such cancer had developed.

The news was so startling that Dr. Alexander Langmuire, the well-known epidemiologist, announced in the *New England Journal of Medicine* that the discovery was of "great scientific importance" and, according to the story by Lawrence Altman in the New York *Times*, added: "Physicians must think more seriously before administering any drug to a pregnant woman."

In spite of all this activity, it was not until late 1971 that the FDA finally issued another weak and ineffectual warning.

All through the spring of 1971, the same monotonous pattern kept repeating itself: the pressure of industry lobbyists to permit the manufacturers to do anything they pleased, as long as it led to profits; the strangely benign condoning of this attitude on the part of the Nixon administration and the highest echelons of the HEW, especially the FDA, the Federal Trade Commission, the Department of Agriculture, and the Department of Justice, to whom cases against industry had to be referred.

Against this coalition, those concerned with genuine consumer protection across the country, led by Ralph Nader, Jim Turner, Dr. Richard Burack, Senators Gaylord Nelson, Warren Magnuson, Abraham Ribicoff, Philip Hart, and others, and Congressmen L. H. Fountain, Benjamin Rosenthal, John Blatnik, and Florence Dwyer, among many, were assembling their tattered troops against their well-heeled adversaries. It would be safe to add that they were joined by most of the scientific and technical personnel of the FDA, the Department of Agriculture, and the Federal Trade Commission.

All the activity, the controversy, the speeches, the polemics, and the incantations pointed inexorably toward one thing: If the consumer wanted any real, as opposed to verbal, protection, there would have to be a reordering of priorities, beginning with the breaking up of the love affair between Nixon and his men with big industry and ending with a realistic strengthening of the Food and Drug Administration with both budget and manpower so that it could pretend to do its job. The total budget for the FDA's nationwide assignment is $20,000,000 *less* than New York City's local Department of Health. For the price of a half a dozen bombers, the FDA's effectiveness could be doubled.

4

The Beautiful Two-Layer Tablet

ONE DAY in the mid-1960's, a six-year-old boy came down with the kind of thing all children go through constantly and naggingly: a virus cold, a sore throat, a slight fever. The family doctor prescribed a regular course of the Parke, Davis wonder drug Chloromycetin. After a spell of several months, the boy developed some unusual-looking black-and-blue marks over his body. The doctor took a blood count. It was leukemia. The boy died within eight months.

During the 1950's, a five-year-old girl, Marilyn, also suffered slightly over her short span of years with the usual sore throats, colds, and minor fevers. Her doctor generously provided her with an ample supply of Chloromycetin on most of these occasions. It wasn't too long before tests began to show that her bone marrow was well on its way to being destroyed, along with her ability to manufacture proper blood. She died nine weeks after this was discovered.

In the same decade, a thirty-eight-year-old woman underwent a six-week treatment with Chloromycetin, after which she developed a marked pallor. The diagnosis was hypoplastic anemia, induced by the Chloromycetin treatment. It took about eight years for her condition to worsen, with occasional blood transfusions to attempt to restore red-cell production and her fading health. By May, 1966, the patient became ghostly pale and incoherent, with marked purpura (bleeding under the skin). There was also evidence of congestive heart failure and a severe neurologic deficit related to brain hemorrhage. The bone marrow specimen was almost totally replaced by myeloblasts. She died shortly after admission to the hospital. The diagnosis was chronic aplastic anemia, induced by Chloromycetin treatment.

A sixty-one-year-old woman from Boston was always in good health, except that she was plagued by a constant series of head colds. Her doctor suggested taking four Chloromycetin capsules a day "at the first sign of a sniffle." Over a period of about a year, she took a total of some sixty capsules, more or less as a prophylactic measure against other colds. The capsules worked. But hypoplasia and myeloblastic leukemia soon developed. Even though the Chloromycetin was discontinued, the patient died fourteen months after the diagnosis was made.

Chloromycetin, known generically as chloramphenicol, was developed in the late 1940's at Yale University, under a grant from Parke, Davis. After the success of penicillin, dozens of pharmaceutical houses had begun screening soil molds of every type in a search for other antibiotics. Parke, Davis' gamble paid off. Out of the Yale research came a drug to battle typhoid fever to a standstill, when no other antibiotic stood a chance.

It was a potent antibiotic. When Parke, Davis brought it out in 1949, it was cheered heartily as a broad-spectrum drug. There was no question that it worked with typhoid fever, Rocky Mountain spotted fever, and a rare urinary tract infection, where other antibiotics failed. Parke, Davis had a hot patent, and it knew it.

The other elegance of Chloromycetin was that, at first, it was thought that it brought about no serious side effects. But before long, in the early 1950's, strange things began happening to patients who used the drug. They began coming down with serious blood disorders, and some of them were fatal. The medical fraternity and the FDA began weighing whether its benefits outweighed its risks.

Its value in the serious but limited diseases like typhoid and Rocky Mountain spotted fever was indisputable. For this reason alone, the drug had very real value, even at the risk of bringing on aplastic anemia or possibly fatal blood dyscrasias, tantamount to drug-induced leukemia. But conservative professional estimates of the number of people who would need Chloromycetin came to some 10,000. For these the drug could be a godsend.

The danger lay in the temptation of the physician to prescribe it for other diseases, although there were plenty of other antibiotics available for these, most of them highly effective.

By June, 1952, the FDA discontinued certification of Chloromycetin on the basis of a nationwide survey. It showed 177 cases of serious blood disorders, all known to be associated with Chloromycetin treatment. Half of these were fatal. Unreported cases would never be known.

In August, 1952, a special committee of the National Academy of Sciences (packed with medical academicians with strong drug industry financial ties) recommended that the drug could be recertified if a sufficiently clear warning label was used in the package insert.

With the warning label, mild as it was, the use of Chloromycetin dropped sharply. But then the Parke, Davis detail men and advertising department got to work. The detail men were told to tell the busy and preoccupied doctors that Chloromycetin had received a blanket clearance from the National Academy of Sciences special committee, and from the FDA too (which was untrue). Sales began climbing. By 1955, Parke, Davis took it on themselves to petition the FDA to soften the warning label. This was refused.

In December, 1959, a Parke, Davis detail man made the mistake of calling on an FDA doctor who had a limited private practice, along with his duties with the FDA. The detail man pointed out boldly that Chloromycetin created no more danger of blood dyscrasias than any other antibiotic.

When called on the carpet for this, Parke, Davis pretended to be shocked and claimed this was strictly against company policy.

Another ominous sign began to show up. National statistics showed that when Chloromycetin came on the market, the number of deaths from aplastic anemia began soaring. When the drug was tabled during the NAS study, the deaths from that disease dropped. When sales again began climbing, deaths from aplastic anemia did likewise.

Consistently, persistently, actively, knowingly, over many, many years, Parke, Davis lured, encouraged, badgered doctors to prescribe the drug, so that prescriptions were pouring into the pharmacies for the treatment of sore throats, colds, acne—even hangnail. Expert medical testimony has indicated that 90 to 99 percent of the prescriptions for Chloromycetin have been for cases for which the drug should never be used.

Instead of being prescribed for 10,000 to 20,000 critically ill people a year, nearly 4,000,000 were receiving the drug. (The main disease Chloromycetin attacks is typhoid fever. There are fewer than 1,000 cases a year in the United States.) Elderly people, those over sixty-five, paid out over $3,350,000 for it.

At its peak, Chloromycetin is reported to have accounted for just about one-third of all of Parke, Davis' profits. Roughly, its cost is almost $20 per 100 capsules. If the 10,000 patients for which the drug might properly be prescribed took 100 tablets a year each, the gross income for the product would be $200,000. If the estimated 4,000,000 receiving the drug through overprescription (risking their lives as they did) each took the same amount, the gross income for the drug would be $80,000,000.

The manner in which Parke, Davis hoodwinked its customer-doctors is a graphic case history of venality. In 1951, an ad in a professional journal touted Chloromycetin for its "uniformity . . . reliability . . . broad spectrum . . . well-tolerated" qualities. It went on to say its topical cream form showed rapid clinical improvement for many superficial infections and dermatological conditions—with no warning whatever.

In 1953, another ad pushed the drug for its broad-spectrum uses "against a great variety of infectious disorders."

The ad also noted "its exceptional tolerance as demonstrated by even mild signs and symptoms of gastrointestinal distress and other side effects in patients receiving the drug." For the first time now, a warning sneaks in at the bottom of the copy: ". . . the broad clinical effectiveness of Chloromycetin has been established, and serious blood disorders following its use are rare. However, it is a potent therapeutic agent, and should not be used indiscriminately or for minor infections— and, as with certain other drugs, adequate blood studies* should be made when the patient requires prolonged or intermittent therapy."

This gracious warning gesture was far from voluntary. The 1952 study by the NAS committee demanded that the warning be given, and even then it was a most inadequate admonition. All through the 1950's the ads continued, and sales soared. Since the drug was effective orally, physicians found it convenient to prescribe for children, and Parke, Davis goaded them on with an ad about its liquid form of Chloromycetin with the headline: "THEY NEVER MAKE FACES AT SUSPENSION CHLOROMYCETIN PALMITATE" . . . pleasant-tasting broad-spectrum antibiotic preparation for pediatric use.

"When you prescribe SUSPENSION CHLOROMYCETIN PALMITATE for your young patients," the ad continued, "therapeutic response is rarely marred by missed doses or spilled doses. Children really like the taste of this custard-flavored preparation. And it slips soothingly down the sorest throat . . . keeps without refrigeration, a convenience appreciated by mothers."

Just how much the parents of the two children mentioned earlier appreciated this convenience will never be known. One physician, Dr. Albe M. Watkins, whose own son died from aplastic anemia caused by Chloromycetin, said: "I do not know of one single victim who would not be alive today had he only been permitted to get well by himself, by nature, without the use of this antibiotic."

---

* Later evidence showed that blood studies were often less than useless, because bone marrow disintegration would not be revealed and even early signs of blood damage might be irreversible.

Others also would not appreciate Parke, Davis' huckstering. They would no doubt include the California woman who was disfigured after taking the drug for an infection that followed the extraction of several teeth, even though she did collect $180,000 in damages before she died. Her claim on which the court made the award was that Chloromycetin had so disfigured her that friends could not recognize her, that she had to shave daily, that she grew a "buffalo hump." About 75 percent of the cases of aplastic anemia developing from Chloromycetin were fatal—a fact you won't find in the Parke, Davis medical journal advertising.

Dr. William Dameshek, a leading hematologist who has since died, clearly stated his opinion in the *Journal of the American Medical Association* in 1960:

> In one month recently, I saw 4 new cases of aplastic anemia. . . . There was no history of the use of other antibiotics or potentially toxic drugs and since the anemia and other manifestations appeared a few months after the last administration of chloramphenicol, it seemed clear that this drug was responsible for the marrow aplasia. . . . The tragic thing about most of these seriously ill cases, most of whom died, is *that the drug need never have been given.* [The italics are the doctor's.]

The testimony of Dr. Albe Watkins is one of the most poignant. He told Senator Gaylord Nelson's hearing into the matter:

> With reference to Chloromycetin (chloramphenicol) Parke, Davis completely omitted any report of toxicity for at least 16 to 18 months. This complete disregard of basic morality was directly responsible for my son's death. Later, when forced to mention possible reactions, they played down any such reports or insisted, as they did at AMA conventions, that there was not any proof of Chloromycetin causing death. They insisted that other medications had been taken concurrently as iron, aspirin, etc., for a long time.
>
> This drug was given me by a representative of Parke, Davis. And I have made it a habit, when they [the detail men] come in

to extol the virtue of the drug, to ask them about the reactions first. And this man told me there were no reactions. This was a perfectly safe antibiotic. So I took the drug home and placed it in my medicine cabinet.

A few days later my son suffered a urinary tract infection, and I went to the cabinet and I looked at the drugs I had. I picked up a bottle of sulfa, and I said, I don't want to give him this, because this might depress his blood-making system, his hemopoietic system. Imagine that. And I looked at Aureomycin and Terramycin, and I said, sometimes this upsets the stomach, and I don't want him to get sick with the drug.

And then I spotted the Chloromycetin. And I gave him the Chloromycetin, which caused his death several months later.

A druggist, about 2 blocks from my office, asked me, "How did you happen to give him Chloromycetin?" This was in 1952. And I said, "This was the one drug that I thought was harmless."

The pharmacist told me, "I told that representative 3 days before that the drug was harmful, that a lady had died in Pasadena"—which was about 3 miles away from my office. So the representative of Parke, Davis knew at the time he gave me the drug; he deliberately lied to me that the drug was harmless.

And as I said, I went home and some days later gave it to my son, and that was the cause. . . .

It is my opinion that Parke, Davis was not nearly as interested in finding out why the drug was toxic as it was in stifling criticism.

In a letter to Parke, Davis written while his son was dying, Dr. Watkins told the company about its advertising and detail-man claims of "no evidence of intolerance," "no untoward effects with these children," and other claims. Regarding his ultimate, fatal decision to use Chloromycetin for his son, he wrote the company:

I might have done better had I taken a gun and shot him—at least he wouldn't have suffered. . . .

I would like to see the directors of this reputable company sit by this little fellow's bedside, see his worried expression and try to explain to him what happened. I would like for the learned scientist who developed this "harmless" drug to give him every one of his 150 shots, as I've had to do—lay awake night after night, watching his every movement, wondering why it had to happen and praying asleep and awake to find it was a bad dream, and James is as healthy and fine as ever.

James died. And he was not the only doctor's son who suffered that fate. Dr. H. A. Hooks, of Texas, lost his seven-and-one-half-year-old son ". . . from aplastic anemia, due in the opinion of 5 specialists, including the State's outstanding hematologist, who attended him," Dr. Hooks writes, "to the routine administration and dosage of Parke, Davis' Chloromycetin (chloramphenicol) by me for an ear-throat infection on *the advice of* representatives of Parke, Davis who repeatedly assured me of its safety, and urged its use *routinely* in general practice. Almost simultaneously, there were 2 other deaths in this area, a child and an adult, which appear to be attributable to the same cause."

The death of the Hooks child took place in 1961, and by this time the FDA belatedly had begun to clamp down on Parke, Davis advertising and package inserts to include a stiffer warning. Over a great deal of protest from the company, the warning was required to be boxed by a printed border and read in part: "Serious and even fatal blood dyscrasias, aplastic anemia . . . are known to occur after the administration of chloramphenicol . . . it is essential that blood studies be made after treatment with the drug. . . ."

It didn't take too long for Parke, Davis to get around this inconvenience to the healthy promotion of the overprescribed drug. It simply ran full-page "billboard" ads in the medical journals, with a large picture of a physician writing a prescription and a headline like: WHEN IT COUNTS—CHLOROMYCETIN (CHLORAMPHENICOL). (The warning still remained in the U.S. package inserts, however—little read and rarely seen.)

And as the sales soared, as the money poured in, as the victims continued unwittingly to trade a sore throat for a case of aplastic anemia or leukemia, Parke, Davis crowed loudly to its stockholders. The drug trade newsletter *The Pink Sheet* commented:

> Parke, Davis Chairman Harry Loynd at April 19th stockholders meeting predicted another $70 million Chloromycetin year for 1966 despite the expiration in October of the product patent, the first basic one on the drug. Even after October, it will be illegal for anyone to manufacture Chloromycetin in the U.S. A key process patent doesn't expire until July, 1967.

Another $70,000,000 year—and uncounted people dying. However, the inevitable did happen in 1967, and Parke, Davis began its campaign to keep Chloromycetin to itself. As Dr. Richard Burack wrote later in his *New Handbook of Prescription Drugs*:

> Parke, Davis's patent on chloramphenicol expired two years ago [1967], and several manufacturers of generic drugs promptly marketed capsules of it, although we did not need any more of this drug on the market than we already had. . . . Parke, Davis discovered that some of the generic capsules therefore did not deliver up their contents to the blood stream as readily as theirs, *the only proved instance to date* where a generic preparation failed significantly to give the same biological effect (i.e., blood level) as a "brand." The Pharmaceutical Manufacturers Association chose to make a celebrated case of the incident. For Parke, Davis that was a mistake, because Senator Nelson and his staff then exposed the tremendously indiscriminate amount of Chloromycetin prescribing that was taking place. National attention was focused on the issue, and doctors got the point.

They got the point, but not until after a long struggle and battle between Senator Gaylord Nelson, the Pharmaceutical Manufacturers Association, and Parke, Davis.

Things had reached such a state in the beginning of 1967 that Dr. James Goddard, Commissioner of the FDA during most of the Chloromycetin extended crisis, said: "I am at my wit's end as to how to stop the medical profession from misprescribing this drug."

The moral grounds were shifting here, away from the irreparable harm Parke, Davis' blatant promotion of a dangerous drug had done. The situation now became an industry infight to keep smaller drug companies from producing an equivalent-value product at an inevitably lower cost, since Parke, Davis had to give up its seventeen-year-long monopoly. The issue was what was missing in the required information supplied by Parke, Davis for other drug companies to produce chloramphenicol after the patent had expired.

Senator Nelson stated that the heart of the matter was that USP (U.S. Pharmacopoeia) standards were the best in the world and that every generic drug had to meet them—yet they could still sell them far under the price that the brand-name companies were selling them. He quoted one case where a hospital was paying a wholesale price of $167 per thousand for a brand-name type of cortisone drug, while an exactly comparable generic name drug cost only $6 per thousand.

But as the hearings proceeded, the Pharmaceutical Manufacturers Association and Parke, Davis pushed Senator Nelson to the limit, and the discussion finally reverted back to the damage Chloromycetin had brought about over the years. Referring to a Parke, Davis ad of 1960 about its "true broad-spectrum coverage" and the very mild warning that accompanied it, Senator Nelson told Dr. Leslie Lueck, director of quality control for Parke, Davis: "There is nothing here that would scare anybody. Your claim was for a potent therapeutic agent and because certain blood dyscrasias had been associated with its administration, you simply said that the drug should not be used indiscriminately."

Then Senator Nelson pointed out a 1967 ad with the new required warning about *"serious, and even fatal blood dyscrasias,"* and asked Dr. Lueck: "How do you explain that you knew how serious these effects could be 10 years ago, and yet in 1960 you were running an ad that did not call this sharply to the attention of the doctor, but then, suddenly, 7 years later, you were running this ad?"

Dr. Lueck explained that both Parke, Davis and the FDA thought that the warning was adequate.

"Do you really mean to tell me, Doctor," Senator Nelson asked, "that you think this first ad says the same thing as the second ad? Do you really mean to say that?"

"I am not saying they say the same thing," said Dr. Lueck.

"Do they give the same warning?" Senator Nelson asked.

"Yes," replied Dr. Lueck, "I think they give the essential warning."

"Let's read it again," said Senator Nelson. "I think this is preposterous."

At this point, Lloyd Cutler, special counsel for the Pharmaceutical Manufacturers Association, cut in. "Mr. Chairman," he said. "I hope I will not sound impertinent, but may I ask what this has to do with the evidence Dr. Lueck has submitted with regard to the evidences of differences of therapeutic brands?"

"I can give you several answers," said Senator Nelson sharply, "but I will give you one that ought to satisfy you. If quality control is important, and I think it is as important as you say it is in the production of drugs for the market place, *quality control of advertising* is just as important. . . .

"I think quality control in advertising is as important as quality control in the production of a drug. That is exactly what I am getting at.

"Now, I will read the two ads again. I will let the public judge this one. You tell me if they both tell the doctor the same thing, and I am going to ask the doctors who testify what their opinion is. We will put into the record the opinion of distinguished doctors on this question. And, if you want to, you can select a number of doctors to appear on this question."

The Senator went on to repeat the wording of the mild warning of 1960. Then he said: "If the doctor reads that, is there anything in there to alert him that there have been deaths indirectly attributed to this drug? If you knew 10 years ago what you know today, why in 1967 do you have a severe warning boxed in heavy print?"

Dr. Lueck protested that the second warning was a duplicate of the package insert (which is hardly ever read or even seen by the doctor), but he did agree that it was a stronger warning. He also repeated that the FDA had approved the ad.

Senator Nelson reacted strongly. "Let me say at this point that I do not have any higher opinion of the FDA's judgment in permitting this kind of advertising than I do of the company's running this ad. I do not think it protects you any to come up and say the FDA approved of a lousy ad. Most of the industry is attacking the FDA most of the time, anyway."

As the hearing went on, more damaging facts began to emerge. Ads continued, without printed warnings, even two years after the NAS special committee's statement about side effects.

But most alarming were the instructions given by Parke, Davis to its detail men. They were to literally memorize and tell to the doctor the following—word for word:

> Intensive investigation by the Food and Drug Administration carried on with the assistance of the Special Committee of eminent specialists appointed by the National Research Council [an arm of the NAS] resulted in unqualified sanctions of continued use of Chloromycetin for all conditions for which it had been previously used.

No mention of the serious blood disorders leading to leukemia. No attempt to warn and inform the doctor of what might really happen. No attempt to keep the drug confined to the 10,000 or 20,000 possible cases where it could be useful—*if* other milder antibiotics failed.

The letter from Parke, Davis accompanying the instructions to be memorized was equally revealing. It said:

> So physicians are of the opinion that Chloromycetin has been taken off the market or that it is just restricted. So physicians have formed the impression that this antibiotic has been associated with the development of blood dyscrasias in large numbers of patients, and will be amazed when you point out the facts.

Hardly able to control his anger, Senator Nelson told the representatives of Parke, Davis and the Pharmaceutical Manufacturers Association: "If you will look at the history of this one, the FDA did not protect the public at all. It is a shocking case. The FDA's actions should not be the defense on which the company stands. The pharmaceutical industry has been a great American industry which has made a great contribution to the health and welfare of the people of this country and I trust will continue to do so. But if they continue with this kind of shoddy practice, I might say to you quite frankly, the industry is going to run into some tough regulations."

He continued by saying he didn't believe *anyone* could read about the instructions to the detail men without thinking that the company was doing its best to avoid giving the doctor the information that blood dyscrasias could occur as a consequence of the use of Chloromycetin and that it should be used only in very serious cases.

But the story does not end here. It grows worse.

Pressed by Senator Nelson, Parke, Davis' Dr. Lueck admitted that the early 1961 advertisements were inadequate in their warnings and that Parke, Davis would not run any such ads like these again, especially after the stronger warning was now required by the FDA.

Dr. Lueck told the Senator that he could assure him that Parke, Davis would print what was on the package insert nearly verbatim, as was done in a February 20, 1967, advertisement.

At this point, Senator Nelson pulled out a copy of a Parke, Davis ad in a British medical journal running just a few days before the model ad Dr. Lueck had praised so highly.

The 1967 British ad was the same old story as 1961. *No warning whatever.* "Clinically unexcelled . . . well-tolerated . . . rapidly absorbed . . . outstanding efficacy in a wide variety of bacterial, viral, and rickettsial infections. . . ."

Not one word about aplastic anemia, fatal blood dyscrasias, leukemia.

Dr. Lueck attempted to explain it. He said: "I would like

to comment that the medical feeling and impressions on the warning requirements on Chloromycetin are different in every country of the world. Parke, Davis & Co. has always met all the requirements, the legal requirements of whatever country we distributed our products in and we have met the necessity of the medical profession in that country. These ads, so far as I know, met all the requirements."

"Well," asked Senator Nelson, "the effect of the drug is the same on people in other countries as it is here, is it not?"

"Largely," Dr. Lueck replied.

"Do you know of some differentiation?"

"Yes," said Dr. Lueck, "there are some minor differentiations but for the sake of this discussion, let us say they are the same."

After an interruption by Attorney Cutler, protesting that all the ads in the British journal had to meet its requirements, Senator Nelson snapped: "So you mean to testify that your company will stand on the proposition that we will send drugs to Tanganyika [now Tanzania], we will send to Latin American countries, we will send drugs to all the underdeveloped countries of the world, and since they do not have any standards, we will fool them all we can and make a great big profit and never tell the doctors that there is a risk of serious blood dyscrasias. Is that what you are telling this committee?"

Attorney Cutler protested that the British doctors were sophisticated, adding that Senator Nelson was indicting every drug company in Great Britain and the United States.

Senator Nelson replied: "Your testimony is that you will meet the standards of the country in which you are advertising, not the standards of safety which the witness has testified is a proper standard, the proper ad which gives this warning that is put in ads in this country. But in countries where the people do not know any better, where the country is *not* protected by laws, you will tell us that you have no compunction about running an ad that will fool a doctor, as you did in California in 1961. . . . I would think that you would not sleep at night—you or any drug company that would do

that. . . . If this is the standard of ethics by which the industry operates, I tell you, you fellows are in for some sad trouble. I do not think this country will stand for it."

Again, if the story could stop here, it would be well. But it
cannot. Because what Senator Nelson did not have on hand
at the time of the hearings were samples of the medical promotion and labeling Parke, Davis was running in Italy and
Japan. There the laws are more lax even than in Great Britain.

The Italian label for Chloromycetin read:

> The fact that therapy with Chloromycetin is remarkably
> without secondary reactions is significant. The preparation has
> been tolerated well by both adults and infants. In the few cases
> in which reactions have occurred, they have been generally lim-
> ited to slight nausea or diarrhea, and their severity rarely re-
> quires suspension of treatment.

Again, *not one word* about the terrifying, creeping blood diseases. Not even a suggestion.

And in Japan? Here Parke, Davis outdid itself, far and
free from the eye of the all-too-gentle FDA watchdog.

For Parke, Davis to confine the recommendations for the
use of Chloromycetin to the very limited, serious diseases it
should be reserved for (and then only after everything else
has failed) would be to cut down on that important Asian
sales market. So the Parke, Davis instructions to the Japanese doctors heartily supported the use of Chloromycetin for:
measles, influenza, syphilis, mumps, colitis, and chicken pox.
No Japanese doctor is asked to weigh the bargain here
against fatal anemias or leukemia—he doesn't even know
about them from the Parke, Davis literature.

And the final *coup de grace* comes with the lyrical description of the drug that Parke, Davis offered the Asian sensibili-
ties of the Japanese medical men: "Chloromycetin," reads
the copy, "is a beautiful, two-layer tablet, sepia on one side,
yellow on the other."

5

The Case of the Missing Monkeys

IT WOULD be refreshing to say that the Parke, Davis Chloromycetin case was atypical of the "ethical" drug business. Unfortunately, it is not. Its pattern is repeated constantly. Parke, Davis has had problems with other products. Many of the friendly competitors that make up the medieval organization of the Pharmaceutical Manufacturers Association have matched these inglorious activities at frequent intervals. There is always the danger of another thalidomide tragedy striking again, and that story is worth examining in the 1970's in perspective.

It was no fault of the drug companies that thalidomide did not strike this country with the tragic wave of phocomelic births that swept across Europe; 5,000 to 6,000 babies were born in less than half a decade with useless stubs for arms and legs or simply flippers where arms should be. The tragedy had one grimly beneficial effect. It shocked Congress into revising the 1938 food and drugs laws and reinforced at least the potential powers of the FDA, as the 1962 amendments went into effect.

It was the William S. Merrell Company, a merger brother of Vick Chemical, that so enthusiastically petitioned the FDA to market thalidomide, as the wonder sleeping pill of all time. Everything about the drug was incredibly soothing and reassuring. Sleep came swiftly on the wings of calmness. In West Germany, where the drug was born in 1953, it swept

across Europe in a wave of popularity unmatched at the
time. A heavy overdose could not be fatal, and side effects
seemed nonexistent. It came out in Europe under many
trade names: Contegran, Disaval, Sotenon, Talimol. The
Merrell Company chose the name Kevadon in 1960 and presented the FDA with volumes of scientific data to support its
request to market the drug here.

The job to check out the data went to the now-famous Dr.
Frances O. Kelsey, of the FDA's Division of New Drugs. She
set out to review the material and verify its safety claims.

There were several things that seemed incomplete to Dr.
Kelsey, and a routine request went out to Merrell to supply
further information. While this was being studied, many doctors and hospitals were permitted to use the drug experimen-
tally. In Britain, without the restraint of an FDA, the drug
was selling as fast as it was in all of Western Europe—some of
it over the counter, without prescription. The medical advertising, typically, punched across the "safety" theme with un-
fettered enthusiasm.

By February, 1961, the incidence of phocomelia had
climbed to three times its normal rate in Germany. No one
tacked the blame on thalidomide. But Dr. Kelsey noted a letter in a British medical journal in which a doctor asked if the
tingling fingers of some of his patients might be tied in with
their use of the drug. Dr. Kelsey brought this to the Merrell
Company's attention and again asked for more information
before she would clear the drug for regular distribution.

Without the FDA, weak as it was under the old 1938 laws,
thalidomide would have been saturating the United States
through the Merrell Company's largesse, just as it was doing
in Europe. In England, any drug company could put any of
its drugs on the market without pretesting it at all. No
agency independent of the manufacturers existed.

The Merrell Company was smarting under the FDA's and
Dr. Kelsey's obstinate refusal to rush through an approval on
thalidomide. At the same time the British manufacturer was
beginning to fight off medical observation that thalidomide
was "fast becoming one of the commonest causes of neuropa-

thy in neurological clinics," according to a letter from the Whipps Cross Hospital to the *British Medical Journal.*

In Germany, preliminary studies began to confirm what was already suspected: Thalidomide was a velvet villain. Of all the mothers who came to his clinic with children born with flippers for arms and grossly stunted legs, 20 percent had been taking thalidomide during pregnancy. Then the doctor interviewed the mothers again. This time half of them now recalled taking the drug. Many of them felt that this was "too innocent a drug to mention" in the first interviews.

After this suspicion came the confirmation. All over Europe, the deformities of thousands of children were shown to be clearly related to thalidomide. The Merrell Company withdrew its application, and thanks to Dr. Kelsey, only a few mothers, who had taken the drug in testing programs, suffered the fate of the Europeans.

The Chief Medical Officer in England wrote: "The tragic results of the use of thalidomide in pregnancy were not due to any failure to apply tests of toxicity generally accepted at the time, but they have naturally given rise to a general feeling that there should be stricter control over the toxicity testing and chemical trial of all new drugs."

As in past history, it took a tragedy of this magnitude to accomplish several things. It pointed to the necessity and urgency of looking beyond immediate, apparent safety, even unto the next generations. It showed that the importance of controlling the *advertising* claims of drugs was as critical as assuring the safety and effectiveness of the drug itself. And it . swept the 1962 amendments triumphantly through Congress. Now the resistant members of the archaic Pharmaceutical Manufacturers of America would face FDA inspection and would have to assume the burden of the proof of both the safety and the effectiveness of a drug. For the first time, the burden of the proof would have to be on the manufacturer. (Today, still, cosmetics, toiletries, and medical devices elude this requirement, and that is why many FDA experts worry about the "time bomb" factors in these areas.)

Most important: Records, reports, clinical and animal

studies under controlled testing were required before a drug could be marketed. But, again, the old question of whether it was possible for the fox to look after the chickens came up. And the same William S. Merrell Company, which was saved by the FDA's intractable stance against thalidomide, comes into sharp focus as an example of what the public faces when the rakish and saturnalian impulses of the drug companies come into play.

The drug was called MER/29, in honor of the first three letters of the manufacturer's name, presumably. Merrell put in a new drug application to the FDA on July 21, 1959. The drug was designed to lower cholesterol levels, since high levels are supposed by some to be dangerous to cardiac and hypertensive patients. Other medical men disagree. They do not feel that cholesterol has been proved to cause or aggravate atherogenic (arteriosclerotic, pulpy deposits on the walls of the arteries) conditions. Regardless of that, which the FDA did not argue with, the agency felt that the application was rather incomplete, especially the evidence for safety in the use of the drug. Again, as with thalidomide, it was suggested that Merrell complete both a one-year study, and a three-month study, with dogs to prove out some of the safety claims.

The Merrell Company did not take too kindly to the delay imposed on them. The assistant to the director of research wrote the FDA to say that the animal tests submitted with the new drug application showed an "exceptionally good" margin of safety for the drug. He pointed out that a study of laboratory monkeys was especially convincing in this regard.

Merrell did, however, begin and continue other animal tests, protesting again that the significance of the monkey tests was being entirely overlooked by the FDA as an indicator of the drug's safety. One FDA medical officer said: "There was little margin of safety for the drug. I indicated my serious concern about the safety and use of such a drug for reducing blood cholesterol. . . . My recommendation was that the application should not be approved in the absence of satisfactory results from extensive, well-controlled clinical studies in which individuals received the drug for a period of several years."

But Merrell kept talking about those monkey tests. The company insisted the tests had shown a total absence of toxicity, and since monkeys were closer to the human being than any other animal, this should bear great weight. The FDA was not at all happy about the rat and dog tests either, where funny things were happening to gall bladders, livers, the corneas of the eyes, gonads, and hair, which seemed to fall out after treatment. The horror symptom of Parke, Davis' Chloromycetin began to show up in the animals in the form of blood dyscrasias for MER/29. But the reports submitted by Merrell miraculously seemed to shift the blame for these conditions onto other things. Somehow, the rat and dog tests seem to have come out with just enough lack of bad evidence to slip by.

By April, 1960, the FDA informed Merrell that its application would be approved on a conditional basis. However, tests would have to be continued. Merrell agreed and began to assemble its big-sales artillery.

One big salvo came with an interdepartmental memo titled "Let's Start Selling," which read in part:

> Let's take a close, critical look at the way we are stimulating the field force on MER/29. Very frankly, I have seen almost nothing going out of here in the way of good sales promotion ideas. . . . I find no change made in the closing [i.e., closing pitch for detail men to memorize] which asked to put 10 patients on it [MER/29]. Why 10? To me it makes sense to ask a doctor to try a drug on two, three, or possibly five patients, but if we're going above that, why not ask for all of them? What do you think of a closing that says in effect: "I am sure that you will want to place all of your post-coronary and coronary-prone patients on MER/29."
>
> Admittedly, the above is only one single, short suggestion, but I think we ought to take a fresh look at our whole campaign on MER/29 with the idea of retaining the essential flavor of the introduction, but getting much more positive in order to motivate more doctors to write scripts [prescriptions].

Before, during, and after the time this cheery piece of sales fluff was going out to the brainwashed detail men (who in turn, brainwashed the doctors), other memos and correspondence were making their way in, out of, and around the Merrell Company.

One highly placed executive wrote to another:

> . . . We have had reports from two clinicians that of the first two patients they placed on MER/29, one died at the end of the week from a coronary. This is not written to alarm anybody as we are confident it was independent of the drug. . . . However, on the surface of the record, you can see how bad this looks.

A research doctor in the field reported back to the Merrell Company the following information regarding three patients:

I. W. (*edema*)

9–7–59	(MER/29) medication started
11–17–59	Eyes started to discharge and were swollen shut
11–18–59	Medication discontinued
12–24–59	Medication restarted
1–4–60	Eyes red and discharging again. This continued to some degree until his death

A. O. (*heart trouble*)

5–25–59	Eyes red and watery until end of study
6–3–59	Study ended
9–7–59	Started on medication again
9–15–59	Eyes were discharging along with other complications and medication was discontinued
12–16–59	Restarted on MER/29
1–21–60	Eyes discharging
2–1–60	Eyes were discharging more along with other complications, and medication was discontinued for last time

A.W.

4–20–59	Started on medication
6–1–59	Eyes were a little red and discharging on last week of 6 weeks study

Regarding a research doctor who appeared to be about to come up with a negative report on MER/29, a cynical inter-office memo between two Merrell medical men reads:

> Dr.——— has made a verbal request for $500 to support his continued study on the effects of MER/29. . . . Although it begins to appear that any report from this study may be a negative one, we may find that we are money ahead to keep Dr.——— busy at it awhile longer, rather than to take a chance on his reporting negatively on so few patients. . . .
>
> My personal recommendation is that the grant-in-aid be approved only to keep Dr.——— occupied for awhile longer.

From a California doctor came this inquiry from the field to the Merrell Company:

> I have had some reports back from the different people in the 50's age bracket, who are taking 1 - 250 mg MER/29 per day, and after 2 to 3 months, they have had itching eyelids, little (crusts) in inner corner of eyes. Also one had a 20-vision and says he is getting slightly blurred vision which clears up and then reestablishes itself when the drug is discontinued and then resumed. I have a lady acquaintance who took it for five months and who had always had a good firm head of hair. However, it began to fall out quite heavily and upon discontinuance of MER/29, it became firmly embedded and healthy.
>
> In your research, have you had any experiences like this?

In replies to letters like this, the Merrell Company most often expressed surprise that such things were happening. But all across the country, medical men were discovering such things as dermatitis, falling hair, color change of hair, and loss of the sex drive. In contrast to these gathering clouds, such interoffice memos as these were making the rounds:

"There seems to be a general acceptance of the idea that MER/29 is reaching a sales volume which is worth protecting. . . ."

From a regional man of the Merrell Company in Texas to

the home office: "Dr. K——— also learned of the dentist being treated by Dr. Schultz, as 'being close to death' in a hospital, and had his office telephone all important drug stores to stop filling and refilling his MER/29 Rx until further notice."

From one Merrell executive to another regarding a retainer fee to a Boston physician: "You will recall we had him on a personal retainer amounting to $2,400 per year, payable in two semi-annual installments. If we wish to maintain this relationship, a payment of $1,200 is now due. My own feelings are that we can't afford to chance alienation of H——— just now (perhaps I shouldn't regard this as blackmail). . . ."

Meanwhile, the Merrell salesboys were busy. In the company newsletter *Sales Talk* such paragraphs as these were running:

> *Time* waits for no one—MER/29 is no exception. The "Medicine" section of the latest issue praises MER/29 in an article "Cutting the Cholesterol." This issue will be in the hands of over 3 million persons. Publicity of this kind will send thousands of patients to their doctors asking about MER/29. Make sure they walk out of the offices with prescriptions.

Contrast note—A letter from a detail man in Harrisburg, Pennsylvania, to the Merrell home office:

> . . . a dermatologist mentioned that a side effect that some of his patients might experience is complete alopecia, even of pubic hair. The doctor asked if I would check to see if such was the case or whether it may be strictly a rumor.

From *Sales Talk* again:

> The quick way to get the non-prescriber to use MER/29 is to use every resource you have at your command to show him that he will be benefiting himself and his sick patients in a giant way just as soon as he uses MER/29. That's any doctor's hot button . . . and you must come down on it harder than ever before.

Contrast note—Field man report to Merrell home office regarding a patient of one of the doctors he calls on, where MER/29 had been prescribed:

Symptoms since December 20, 1960:

1. Dry, flaky alligator type skin ichthyosis type with secondary infection, then yeast, mold, monilial type in crotch and inner thighs (before antibiotic).
2. Loss of scalp hair.
3. Hair color change from dark brown to light blond, also eyebrows, etc.
4. Loss of libido.
5. Skin condition such that patient finds it almost impossible to move around and carry out usual work, etc.
6. Patient referred to Dr. H——— who happened to have two more patients whose dermatitis may have been touched off by MER/29. . . .

From *Sales Talk* again—Instructions to Merrell detail men on how to approach the doctor:

First, MER/29 is a proven drug. It has been administered under controlled conditions to more than 2000 patients for periods up to three years. There is no longer any valid question as to its safety or lack of significant side effects. . . .

Contrast note—Intramural memo regarding complaint of FDA's Dr. Talbot:

Dr. Talbot stated that he has been annoyed by letters and personal visits by physicians complaining about MER/29. In each case, the complaint has been based on reports of hepatitis. . . .

From *Sales Talk* again:

We heard 8 words the other day that neatly handle one of your biggest problems. When a doctor says your drug causes a side effect, the immediate reply is: "Doctor, what other drug is the patient taking?" Even if you know your drug can cause the

side effect mentioned, chances are equally good the same effect is
being caused by a second drug. ". . . Doctor, what other drugs
is the patient taking? Been doing it for years? Why didn't you
tell us, then?"

Contrast note—Merrell detail man to home office:

A pharmacist in my territory stated that when taking
MER/29 for about a week or more his eyes started to tear and
burn slightly. When therapy was discontinued these symptoms
disappeared, but upon resuming MER/29 therapy he complained of the same problem. Do you have any information as to
why he might be getting this reaction, if it is possibly from
MER/29?

From *Sales Talk* again:

Here's one that seems like a red hot idea for MER/29 . . . if
it's your style. It's from Tim Bowen, Charlotte, N.C. Aimed particularly at the "wait and see" physician, Tim's close [*i.e.,* final
sales pitch to the doctor] goes something like this (we got it third
hand):

Doctor, I can appreciate and admire your caution about any
new drug, but MER/29 has been on the market almost a year
now and was studied in thousands of patients for years before
that. Its rate of use indicates that acceptance is broadening rapidly. Perhaps these words of Alexander Pope have some bearing
on your consideration of MER/29: "Be not the first by whom the
new is tried, nor the last to lay the old aside."

Lots of power there . . . can your style be bent just a bit to fit?

Contrast note—Merrell interoffice memo:

The FDA wants a statement from us to the effect that we have
supplied all toxicity data in animals and man, including that
available to us from outside sources. The implications here are
obvious, and on pressing Nestor [an FDA executive], he offered
as an example a comment that a Dr. Wong of Howard University [made when he] visited us in April to describe results in
chickens indicating interference with ovulation. Dr. Wong states
we ignored the results, and Nestor declared this could be
grounds for suspension of the NDA [new drug application].

It was hard to tell at the time just what was going on. If the animal tests were all that Merrell had said they were in its new drug application, it was strange that there were so many reports of adverse reactions all over the country. Especially after the monkey tests that Merrell had touted so loudly, since monkeys do approximate the human system so closely.

Perhaps the hyperthyroid Merrell sales managers would have gone on crowing to their hearts' content for a considerably longer time if it had not been for a car pool in Cincinnati, Ohio, that happened to carry Tom Rice, at that time acting chief inspector of the FDA in that area. Carson Jordan, another member of the car pool, knew that Rice worked for the FDA and brought him some particularly interesting information one morning in February, 1962.

Carson's wife, it seemed, had once worked on the animal studies at Merrell for the MER/29 project. In fact, she had been one of the principal technicians involved with the laboratory monkeys. Carson told the FDA inspector as they rode to work that morning that his wife felt sure that the records of the animal studies had been falsified to make them look good. Not only that, but she resigned her job in the animal testing laboratory, because she didn't like the way her superior was running the tests. She also felt very strongly that he would have no qualms about "doctoring" the results.

The Acting Chief Inspector Rice lost no time in interviewing Mrs. Jordan. He learned that she had been in charge of both weighing and dosing the monkeys tested with MER/29 and the control group, those monkeys that received only a sugar placebo. There were three or four in each group.

What bothered her most was the monkey designated as M-34. It seemed very sick to her, and its eyes "did not look right," she told the inspector. It seemed mean, withdrawn, and it continually missed a box it had been trained to jump into. Shortly after this, she was instructed by one of her superiors to falsify the charts. Then she learned that a perfectly healthy monkey that had not been on MER/29 was substituted for the ailing monkey. The healthy monkey weighed about ten pounds more than the sick one. She had to make up the false charts three times, with spurious weights supplied by her superior.

Slowly, the whole story shaped up under the scrutiny of the FDA investigators. The laboratory test monkeys were only the tip of the iceberg. *All* the female rats of one study died before the completion of a six-week observation. In some surviving male rats, adverse blood effects appeared including changes in leukocytes, granulocytes, and lymphocytes—none of these findings were reported to the FDA. Various blood dyscrasias were observed in blood smears taken from monkeys that had been given MER/29; none were observed in the control monkeys. Merrell had tried to change the records so that it appeared that all monkeys were supposed to have had these anomalies. In a dog study, those which had died were replaced by three additional dogs to bolster the statistical figures. Among beagle dogs, Merrell covered up the fact that portions of the gonads had undergone "marked tubular and interstitial atrophy."

Irreparable eye damage to the lab animals, with the lenses of the eyes clouded so much that the retina could not be observed, was covered up. Other eye infections were rampant, foreshadowing the later reports by doctors about their human patients. One pathologist wrote in his report that he had "never seen such an involvement of the lens."

Endless unfavorable reports were suppressed or withheld. Interdepartment memos at the time of the studies contained sentences like these: ". . . You will recall that during our conversation concerning this subject, it was decided that we should at least temporarily refrain from telling Dr. H——— or any other person outside the Merrell organization that MER/29 undergoes rather rapid acid hydrolysis." ". . . We were not thinking here so much of honest clinical work as we were of a pre-marketing softening prior to the introduction of the product."

But even with all this in the background, the Merrell Company's *Sales Talks* kept churning along. As an extra bonus, it presented to the detail men this story:

NEW LOOK FOR MER/29 STOCK PACKAGES

No doubt you've seen the new blue carton for MER/29. . . .
The color coordinated Merrell "look" will lend prestige to the
entire line of Merrell specialties on the pharmacist's shelf.

Aggressive action against the grave misdoings of the pharmaceutical companies seldom comes from the top echelons of
the Department of Health, Education, and Welfare, parent
to the FDA. In fact, there is ample evidence to show how the
conscientious work of FDA scientists and technicians is
blocked constantly at the high administration levels. The
Abbott intravenous fluid case took Nader's prodding to force
the FDA top administration into action. The successful fight
against MER/29 was forced to a crisis by a regional chief inspector. Only a Congressional hearing brought any real
meaning to the fight against the abuses of Chloromycetin. In
the cyclamate story, then-HEW Secretary Finch stalled un-
successfully to keep cyclamates on the market. All of these attitudes reflected by high HEW officials are enough to send a
few shudders up the back of a consumer.

Quite in character with this picture, and illustrative of
high government officials and their irresponsible courtesy to
the drug companies, is the story of Upjohn's antibiotic Panalba.

If it had not been for HEW Secretary Robert Finch's hesi-
tations about providing Congress with legal access to the
FDA files, the Upjohn Panalba story might never have sur-
faced.

In May, 1969, North Carolina's Congressman L. H. Fountain was ready to attack the FDA's lackluster efforts to crack
down on the obvious abuses the pharmaceutical industry was
perpetrating almost daily. He was particularly distressed by
the second Chloromycetin case, involving the intravenous
form of the drug, where the FDA had permitted Parke,
Davis to continue marketing its product with older, less-strict
labeling than that of a new generic competitor.

The focus of attention was on what are called antibiotic

combination drugs. These combine every sort of antibiotic to produce glowing advertising and sales copy to appeal to the doctors. It mattered little if the drug companies were piling up a mass of drugs which all did the same thing for the patient or if there were not enough of each separate ingredient so that the drug became less useful or even hazardous to the patient.

But "combination drugs" were far from useless for the manufacturer. He could give them an appealing brand name and charge outrageously for them. Then he could con the doctors through his advertising and detail men into believing they were giving the patient something extra.

At 10:30 A.M. on May 9, 1969, Congressman Fountain asked Donald Gray, his senior staff investigator, to request from the FDA all the recent files on its review of these combination antibiotic drugs. This is an ordinary, routine request. The FDA told Gray that they would be ready for him within the hour.

But then something unusual happened. Within half an hour, the FDA called Gray back and told him that this routine request had been submitted out of the FDA to HEW Secretary Finch's office. Congressman Fountain could not recall any other time that such a request had been sent over the FDA Commissioner's head to his boss in the HEW for approval.

Gray pushed hard for a reason for this. He was told that there was an unwritten FDA policy about providing files to Congress in "potentially explosive situations." Decisions like this, it was said, could only be made by the Secretary himself. Gray asked for a legal basis for this procedure. He was stalled off until after lunch for an answer.

When no legal basis was supplied by 2 P.M., Gray went personally to the FDA offices. Again, no reason was supplied. Finally, at 3 P.M., Gray learned that Secretary Finch passed the word along down the chain that he could have access to the files.

Technically, the FDA Commissioner has full authority to grant access to a Congressional committee. He also has full authority to decide about the marketing status of a drug, without reference to the HEW Secretary at all.

But when Gray went over the reluctantly released files, it became apparent where the hitch was. It involved the status of Upjohn's antibiotic combination drug Panalba. It quickly became apparent that Secretary Finch, who had no technical training himself, had stepped into the breach to decide whether the drug would be permitted to continue on the market or not in the face of some very disturbing evidence.

The bloodletting came at 3 o'clock, when legal counsel William Goodrich called FDA Commissioner Herbert Ley's office to tell them to give the files to Gray, that all had been cleared.

Later, the Fountain committee learned that representatives of the Upjohn Company, makers of Panalba, had arrived at Secretary Finch's office just four days before all the above convolutions had taken place. The FDA was instructed to "hold up on the matter" as a result of the meeting.

The crux of the problem, as far as the Upjohn Panalba stall was concerned, lay in the fact that the FDA had joined in the opinion of the National Academy of Sciences some five months before that the antibiotic Panalba was simply and purely ineffective as a fixed dosage (tetracycline and novo-biocin) combination. Upjohn had thirty days to send in any new information that would contest this decree, as specified by law. If no information came in from Upjohn, the drug would be removed from the market, again according to law.

But it wasn't a case of Panalba merely being ineffective. A later report from the National Academy of Sciences revealed that the novobiocin portion of the drug showed *"clearly evident imminent hazards to the health of patients."*

Instead of the thirty-day deadline for Upjohn to come up with proof of safety and effectiveness, the FDA kindly extended the grace period for 120 days. The news of the "imminent hazard" factor turned up at the FDA around the end of March. This added a whole new dimension to the case. But it wasn't until a month later that FDA Commissioner Herbert

Ley wrote a letter to Upjohn impressing on the company that the "clearly evident imminent hazards to the health of patients" made action imperative and further stalling out of the question.

The letter was never mailed, but an immediate meeting on the first of May was called with Upjohn officials. The FDA position of Commissioner Ley was clear and unequivocal. It set up these actions:

1. An immediate warning letter to all doctors.
2. Decertifying all stocks of Panalba and any other drug containing novobiocin.
3. Recall of all stocks of such drugs from the pharmacists' shelves, including Panalba and another similar Upjohn product.

Dr. Ley expected controversy with the Upjohn people, and he got it. In spite of the imminent-hazard evidence, Upjohn's president, vice-president and general counsel, director of product research, and outside attorney howled that the FDA was being unreasonable and that most of the steps the FDA wanted to take to protect the public were unnecessary. It was not a happy May Day. When Upjohn's president, Ray Parfet, said he hadn't "seen" the toxicity of the drug in the ten years it had been on the market, Dr. Ley pointed out that there had been confirmed reports of a high frequency of liver problems, to say nothing of the frightening specter of aplastic anemia, blood dyscrasias, high fevers, and rashes.

The protests from the pharmaceutical men were loud and predictable: "The FDA is going beyond the National Academy of Science's recommendation" (it wasn't); the FDA action would be "terribly extreme."

The attorney retained by the company said: "We have not anticipated your drastic and shocking call for cut-off by May 31."

But Dr. Ley remained firm. He warned the Upjohn officials that if the company failed to abide by the FDA recommendations, he would not only cancel certificates but call for multiple seizures. He said, however, that he would give them until the following Monday (May 5) to try to answer the charges and would withhold the press release until that time.

Upjohn was in a spot. It flatly refused to agree with the FDA proposals. It demanded that no press release be issued to inform the doctors and the public about the dangers and inadequacies of Panalba. It demanded that no warning letter be sent to doctors. It demanded the prompt recertification of the drug. It called for a hearing (not required in cases of "imminent hazard") before it would make up its mind about taking the drug off the market.

But the FDA meeting was not the only one the Upjohn executives held that day. They went upstairs, over the heads of the FDA Commissioner's office, and into the welcoming arms of HEW Secretary Finch and his Undersecretary John G. Veneman. The upshot of this meeting was that Veneman picked up the phone, called Commissioner Ley, and told Ley's deputy (Ley was not in at the time) that he ought to do exactly what the Upjohn people wanted. In this way, Upjohn would get free from the uncomfortable process of admitting that Panalba was not only ineffective but was also a clear-cut threat to the health and safety of the people who were using it.

Dr. Ley stuck to his guns. On the day after the phone call from Undersecretary Veneman, he wrote a memo to Veneman's boss expressing his feelings about the matter. He told about Veneman's request to withhold the publicity and warnings about the drug and to let the company go merrily along pawning it off on an unsuspecting public. Then he wrote:

> The basic question before us is whether the Government is prepared to move promptly and effectively to stop the use of a hazardous drug when the available facts and the national drug law dictate such action. We believe that the facts show clearly that Panalba presents serious hazards to patients who take it. . . . When the Food and Drug Administration certifies a stock

of an antibiotic, it certifies that the drug is safe and effective
when used as directed in its labeling. I cannot issue such a certi-
ficate for Panalba. . . . [W]e have the right and the obligation
to move to protect the public by requiring its removal from the
market, and by requiring an appropriate warning to be issued to
the doctors of the Nation. . . .

If the Department [*i.e.*, HEW] is unable to accept this recommendation, I request your instructions as to the departmental
position that I should follow. . . .

With this forceful and uncompromising letter, Dr. Ley included some background information on Panalba: how the
novobiocin component of the drug had been shown to create
a high incidence of adverse reactions, up to 20 percent; how
people who took it rapidly got drug-resistant germs, while
better drugs were available that didn't cause this effect; and
how the patient should not be exposed to novobiocin in order
to get the benefits of tetracycline, the other component of
Panalba.

The decision should have been up to Dr. Ley. But because
of the machinations whirling around both the HEW and the
FDA, it was obvious that he couldn't make it, especially in
the light of Veneman's phone call. Ley could only wait and
see how his recommendation would be received by Secretary
Finch.

Finch, of course, had no expertise whatever in the pharmaceutical profession. The consumer would have a right to
ask why the ultimate decision should be his in such a dangerous situation and in the face of such a strong recommendation by his own commissioner.

But Dr. Ley waited. He did not hear anything until the
morning of May 9, the day all the commotion started. But at
9:15, he was agreeably surprised. The Surgeon General himself issued an order in agreement with Dr. Ley that the drug
must be taken off the market.

But Ley's vindication was short-lived. Within fifteen minutes, he learned that Secretary Finch had decided that the
drug *should* be allowed to remain on the market pending a

hearing, which would take anywhere from one to five years.

Fortunately for the vulnerable consumers of Panalba— thousands of them—this was the morning that Mr. Gray, of Congressman Fountain's office, put in his phone call to request the files. It was the morning that the wires between the FDA and its parent HEW were burning up with questions as to what to do about the request.

By afternoon of that day, Secretary Finch threw in the sponge and permitted Mr. Gray to receive the files. At the same time, Finch reversed his own decision of 9:30 A.M. and decided to go along with Dr. Ley's recommendation to take Panalba off the market. The fight was over at last, thanks to the Fountain committee. And the consumer not only gained safety but saved $20,000,000 a year that had been spent for a worthless and dangerous drug.

Naturally, the question arises: What would Finch have done if the sudden, hot breath of the Congressional investigation had not blasted through the offices? No one will ever know, but it's fairly easy to guess. Under the high leadership of the HEW, fostered by the administration's benevolent and fraternal relationship with the drug companies, the consumer always comes last on the totem pole—if at all.

6

The Uneasy Road to Tranquillity

THE WHOLE great tidal wave of tranquilizers, sedatives, antidepressant pills, analgesics, and other drugs falling roughly within the class the doctors like to call psychotropics has reached an all-time peak, with no end in sight. The present population of 200,000,000 guinea pigs is so massively overprescribed with drugs that dull or kill the senses that Orwell's *1984* or Huxley's *Brave New World* might just become understatements.

Knowledge about what all this is doing to us is skimpy at best. Even the experts don't know, but those who give the situation thought are worried. The market is so flooded with brand names, generic names, mixtures, and combinations that no one has a simple answer, and very few have any reasonable grasp of the problem at all. This is, of course, aside from and in addition to the drug abuse question. The dangers lurking in the legitimate Rx psychological drug business may even be greater. Illegal drug abuse has only one very questionable bright spot: It is actually less extensive today than it was in the early 1900's. At that time the consumers of hundreds of patent medicines were full-fledged opium addicts without even knowing it, except when they couldn't get to the corner drugstore for their opiate-ridden syrups.

But the legitimate prescription traffic today is terrifying. Statistics show that there is little question that we are a drugged society, especially in the psychotropic areas. It is as if millions of us wanted to avoid those moments of normal stress that are part of everyday living and were willing to pay the cost in dullness, apathy, and a collection of very serious side effects and reactions to pay for it. Says the *Medical Letter* (the highly regarded information periodical for physicians) about two specific, well-known tranquilizers:

> . . . there are no reliable figures on the number that do take them, but it is known that few drugs of any class are prescribed more often. Many drugs are vastly overprescribed, and a great number of persons are being led into unhealthy and costly drug dependence by physicians' too-ready acceptance of the therapeutic advice given by a not-disinterested manufacturer.

Said Dr. Richard Pillard, of Boston University: "[this is] part of a trend to suggest the use, both of antidepressants and tranquilizers not only for specific mental illnesses, but to soothe life's ordinary woes."

Dr. Daniel Freedman, of the University of Chicago, told staff economist Ben Gordon, of the Nelson Senate subcommittee: "One thing, I think, we do know in psychiatry is that grief is very important to normal experience, and that stunted emotional working-through of these problems can lead to a serious psychiatric problem. In general we think in psychiatry that trying to meet the challenges, the ups and downs of life, are important to development."

In one recent year, psychotropic drugs totaled 178,000,000 prescriptions—or nearly one prescription for every human guinea pig in the country, adult and child. The consumer paid nearly $700,000,000 for these. None of these prescriptions includes combination drugs, which are those tranquilizers combined with another component. Nor do they include the staggering over-the-counter drug sales used to coddle the nerves or emotions. The figures, according to Dr. Jerome Levine, of the National Institute of Mental Health, show that the prescriptions totaled 1.33 for every adult in the country.

Highest on the charts are the minor sedatives (experts

argue against the free use of the word "tranquilizer"), such as Miltown, which add up to nearly 60,000,000 prescriptions. Next come the hypnotics, such as short-acting barbiturates, with just about 30,000,000 prescriptions. Stimulants, like the amphetamines, account for over 25,000,000. Sedatives, such as the longer-acting barbiturates, come to a little over 20,000,000. Major "tranquilizers," like chlorpromazine, total some 15,000,000, while certain antidepressants come to about 12,000,000.

Under this regimen, it is a wonder that half the population isn't wandering around in a daze. But future storm warnings come from a situation pointed out by Dr. Leo E. Hollister, of the Veteran's Administration Hospital, Palo Alto, California. He notes that in certain school districts in his area, up to 30 percent of the elementary school children have been put on an amphetaminelike pill called methylphenidate by doctors in order to keep them from being overactive. Normally, the drug is supposed to wake people up, but half doses for children have shown it to have the opposite effect. Dr. Hollister's concern is that if such a group of hyperactive children are being drug-oriented in grade school, how can any reduction of drug abuse be anticipated when they reach the critical high school age? To them, drugs are being made as routine as Cheerios.

Since children are normally hyperactive, Dr. Hollister suggests in light irony that it would be better to give the teacher a sedative pill.

None of the complaints of the overdrugged society, however, should reflect on the very real and almost miraculous benefits that the psychotropic drugs have brought about in mental institutions. Less than two decades ago, an institutionalized patient found himself almost literally in the land of the hopeless. In the mid-fifties there were over 500,000 patients in mental hospitals. If the expected rate had continued, there would be nearly 750,000 today. With the help of some of the psychotropic drugs, there are only some 400,000 in these institutions today. Some $5 billion has been saved in patient care, according to National Institute of Mental Health figures.

However, there are two catches. One is that overprescription is hitting a far wider group—so-called normal people—and extending the problem to a far wider population base. Second, the United States pharmaceutical manufacturers have been staking their claims for the inordinately high prices of their brand-name drugs on their research and development costs. Aside from the fact that these costs are swollen by trivial manipulation of molecules for the sake of getting a patent, or getting around one, their track record in initiating breakthroughs in the tranquilizer field has been minuscule.

Chlorpromazine was discovered and developed by the French firm Rhône Poulenc, and the American firm Smith Kline & French that picked up the patent from the French company garnered the questionable honor of getting there first so that it could charge rocket-high prices for it. The United States company promptly put the drug on the market for $32 a thousand capsules. A Canadian company, picking up the same French patent there, was able to sell it for $2 a thousand.

Other variations of chlorpromazine were developed, including triflupromazine, with a British patent passed along to Smith Kline & French. Several other British, French, and Swiss patents caught the American companies flat-footed.

Rauwolfia, which furnished the alkaloid reserpine, was developed by the Swiss firm of CIBA, and a flood of variations of this drug were developed under British and Canadian patents.

A British doctor named Berger began his work on what was to become meprobamate (Miltown and Equanil are the same drug) for the British Drug Houses of England, then came to this country to clean up with Carter Products.* (Carter licensed Wyeth to make Equanil on the condition

* Carter-Wallace (of Carter's Little Liver Pill fame) was too small to "do justice" to the market which Berger, in his writings, encouraged. So he pressured the company into licensing and giving Berger a very significant piece of the action. In fact, the drug is no better than inexpensive phenosorbital and has been demoted from the USP.

that Wyeth slap 20 percent of its revenue into advertising
and promotion.) Librium and Valium, two of the best sellers,
are Swiss developments. The early work on lithium salts was
done by an Australian. Both the National Institute of Mental
Health and the Veterans Administration have made major
contributions to the development and knowledge of the sedatives ("tranquilizers") that are touted to have had such
major impact on the seriously ill psychotic patients who
would have had little help otherwise. The American companies who market many of these foreign developments of questionable worth have shown consistent impulses to charge ra-
pacious prices for them.

According to Henry Steele, of Rice University, Smith
Kline & French found itself without a "mild tranquilizer" to
offer to this hungry market, so they took their potent block
buster, Compazine, designed only for psychotics and packed
full of choice side effects, and pushed it to the hilt by advertising it as a soothing calmer for the tired businessman or
housewife.

The method of advertising used for these escape agents
from the stress of normal living continues to make the professional journals look like an annex of Madison Avenue's worst
attributes. The roots of the massive overdosing of the population can be traced almost certainly to this cause.

Dr. Fritz Freyhan, director of psychiatric research for a
large New York hospital, analyzed a handsome seven-page
brochure of Roche Laboratories for its tranquilizer Valium.
He points out that there are no actual misstatements in the
copy but that it grossly misleads by implication, is full of seductive allusions to preventing crises, coping with life, and
helping therapy to swift success. He calls the advertisement a
"flagrant example of transgressing from truth to fiction" and
urges medical editors to develop greater resistance to this
kind of skilled deception.

The worst flood of "tranquilizing" ads are those which
push the doctors toward prescribing the drugs for every little
up-and-down of normal living. Roche Laboratories will tell
you in one medical journal ad for the doctors that "Sally

Wilson has lost her reputation . . ." and then go on to say
that Sally isn't the grouch she used to be. She doesn't flare up
and lash out at business or at home the way she used to. She's
less tense and taut. She's more friendly and cheerful, and all
that sort of thing. Good for Sally. Good for profits. Good for
Roche. Merck, Sharp & Dohme want the doctors to know
that Elavil HCL will knock the living daylights out of a situation when anxiety accompanies depression, and Wyeth suggests to the doctor that when his patient's work piles up on
the desk, there's nothing better than Serax to get that back-
log out of the way.

Pfizer made sure that the playground and grade school
market is not ignored with a three-page medical journal ad
that shows a tearful little girl and the headline: SCHOOL, THE
DARK SEPARATION, "MONSTERS," and then goes on to extol the
virtues of Vistaril, which will pop a child off to slumberland
before she could say "Pfizer Laboratories."

How does this blatant huckstering get this way? What is
the attitude of the drug company executives when they are
challenged about this sort of antisocial action? A good insight
into a typical case involves the ubiquitous Abbott Laboratories again.

In April, 1970, FDA Commissioner Charles Edwards
rapped Abbott on the knuckles for its advertisement involving its tranquilizing sedative Placidyl that had appeared
in a medical journal. Abbott had falsely claimed superior
values of its product over others in reference to "presleep ex-
citation," "nocturnal confusion and hangover," "physiological response," and "respiratory depression." Further, Commissioner Edwards pointed out to the company that the ad
studiously avoided warning the doctor about the distinct possibility of Placidyl creating blurred vision, profound hypno-
sis, convulsions, and toxic psychosis on withdrawal, plus unusual anxiety, tremor, ataxia (a drunken gait), slurring of
speech, memory loss, perceptual distortions, irritability, agitation, and delirium.

And there were other problems that Abbott didn't bother
to warn the doctors about. They included nausea and vomit-

ing, weakness, dizziness, sweating, muscle twitching, plus confusion and hallucinations from 500 mg. for daytime sedation, to say nothing of transient delirium resulting from this drug in combination with certain others that many patients might also be taking.

To leave these warnings out would seem, even to the layman, to be somewhat discourteous or, at the least, forgetful. Commissioner Edwards was thinking along these lines when he requested that the company discontinue its advertising schedule in short order and run a corrective ad with a boxed-in headline stating: PUBLISHED TO CORRECT A PREVIOUS ADVERTISEMENT WHICH THE FOOD AND DRUG ADMINISTRATION CONSIDERED MISLEADING.

It would almost seem axiomatic that it would be convenient for a doctor and patient to know about all these problems before prescribing or taking Placidyl. Forewarned is forearmed. Then, of course, both could weigh the risk and decide whether to go ahead. Abbott felt differently. The company fought Commissioner Edwards' requests down to the wire. It insisted that the ad did not need to carry each specific adverse symptom and that the ad met all legal requirements. If those are met, who cares about ethical and humanistic requirements, the company might just as well have asked.

Responding to Abbott's contentions, the FDA replied that it was in disagreement with the company's point of view almost in its entirety. "Under the circumstances," the FDA letter to Abbott stated, "we see no advantage in continuing discussions along the lines you suggest. We continue to regard the ad as false and misleading."

As a routine matter in this type of FDA action, arrangements were made for an FDA inspector to collect a sample of Placidyl via the seizure route. In addition he requested an immediate inspection of the Abbott firm to obtain copies of current promotional labeling. Richard Kasperson, then an Abbott vice-president, flatly refused to supply the FDA inspector with the labeling matter. In a shift of mind, however, Abbott later decided to go along with the request. But up until the bitter end, Abbott stated that it did not feel that a remedial ad was warranted. It tried to slip by the corrective ad with a very small headline box regarding the "misleading" aspect of the former ad. But at long last the correction was made so that doctors would have a clear idea about the dangers and side effects of the drug.

This type of activity is taking place constantly throughout the industry. Just about a year later, Ralph Nader and his colleague Jim Turner brought the dangers of the potent Smith Kline & French tranquilizer Stelazine to the attention of both doctors and the public. The drug had been pushed onto 10,000,000 people as a mild sedative (which it wasn't; it was both powerful and dangerous) over the fifteen years it had been on the market. Millions of people were being unnecessarily exposed to such adverse reactions as irreversible drooling, tremors, a shuffling gait, and other symptoms related to dread Parkinson's disease. Jim Turner noted in a speech that a German doctor in 1968 had discovered that 20 to 25 percent of the patients in a mental hospital had come down with serious side effects that would last for many years or perhaps indefinitely.

Turner sharply criticized the FDA for permitting Stelazine to go on the market when it had available a study that showed 43 percent of one test group of patients who came down with symptoms of Parkinson's disease. The FDA, under the Nader-Turner pressure, acknowledged that it was forcing revised labeling of the drug by Smith Kline & French.

If the labeling and advertising for these potent psychotropic drugs (and all prescription drugs, for that matter—after the National Academy of Sciences condemned Panalba, the *Journal of the American Medical Association* accepted a glowing advertisement for it) is so often so misleading, why do the medical journals accept these ads? They are often in contradiction to editorial matter. The economic reason is, of course, obvious. The journals need the advertising revenues in order to exist. But even twinges of conscience seem to be missing from the publishers of these respected journals when it comes

to advertising acceptance. Some would run an ad on one
page and an editorial against the drug on another. As one
doctor told the Nelson Senate subcommittee: "I don't see
how you can inform people on page 22 and misinform them
on page 3."

One well-known doctor said: "Were there a 'Medical
Journal Efficacy Study,' the *Journal of the American Medical Association* and other prestigious journals might be taken off the
market because the toxicity of their advertisements outweighs any advantage to be derived from their textual material."

According to Senator Nelson, the powerful journal of the
AMA testified in 1962 that it was going to stop accepting ads
for fixed combination drugs, such as Panalba. But the ads
continued. "Now I think the public has got a right to be indignant and critical," said the Senator. "What do you expect
the public to think of a profession that won't discipline itself?
All the public is saying is 'For heavens sake, do something
about better prescribing practices.' "

With all this overprescribing, thanks to the persuasive
push of the pharmaceutical companies, the country has
added to its drug abuse problem. Legal prescriptions are providing a substantial base for the cultivation of the drug culture of the day. Children see their parents wash down a Miltown, (Equanil, meprobamate) phenobarbital, Seconal
(Secobarbital), or amphetamine on the slightest excuse and
automatically assume that their own experimentation can't
be much worse than that. As Dr. Stanley Yolles, of the National Institute of Mental Health, said: "The growing dependence on both sleeping pills and stimulants poses an increasing threat to the nation's health. The problem of drug
abuse is increasingly apparent among children at the junior
high level and, because of the potency of fads in early adolescence, the problem begins to affect students in the upper
grades of elementary schools, as well."

There is considerable confusion and misunderstanding on
the part of the layman concerning all this class of drugs that
attempts to deal with psychological problems. Dr. Leo Hol-

lister, of Palo Alto's Veterans Administration Hospital, breaks them down into several classifications.

Antipsychotics are those drugs used for major mental disorders such as schizophrenia. These are the real tranquilizers, not to be confused with the minor forms such as Miltown and Equanil (meprobamate). Chlorpromazine (thorazine) is the leader of the pack in this class. All of these powerhouse drugs carry with them potent and dangerous side effects, such as the ones described for Stelazine. There are about fifteen drugs in this class, under a bewildering variety of both brand and generic names. Anyone who would take one of these drugs for mild depression is risking life, limb, and psyche. Yet, Smith Kline & French didn't hesitate to promote its drugs of this class to the extent that 10,000,000 people took them over the years. Shades of Chloromycetin again: Keep just within the legal bounds, and push like hell. Keep those cards, letters, and prescriptions coming. Keep those labels and ads reading very soft and very smoothly. If the FDA blows the whistle, there will simply be a microfine, in the face of macroprofits.

Antidepressants were developed some years after the chlorpromazine group, although they are chemically related. Known principally as tricyclics, these drugs are prescribed in place of heavy stimulants such as amphetamines, which had previously been the only way of treating depression. They tend to block an enzyme known as monoamine oxidase and are sometimes called MAO inhibitors because of this. (Parnate, a brand name, is a leader in this group.) They are advertised to be effective for treating the lonely despair of older people, who formerly were treated with prolonged hospitalization or electroconvulsive therapy. But this group makes up only about 20 percent of the people who suffer from deep depression. As a result, the tricyclics have been overprescribed to a broad spectrum of other patients, and the results have not been at all good. Not only have they been shown most frequently to be ineffective but downright dangerous. Doctors are warned to try milder forms of treatment first.

Anti-anxiety or sedative drugs are sometimes referred to as the minor tranquilizer group. They include Miltown and Equanil, among others, and have not been shown to be superior to the old-fashioned sedatives phenobarbital or chloral hydrate (the latter is especially safe, according to Dr. Richard Burack). Chemically, however, they differ sharply from the majors. Because anxiety is so common and comes in spurts among normal people, it has never been proved whether these "minor tranquilizers" are any better than plain sugar-pill placebos, dummy medicine. In spite of the fact that patients have indicated a calming effect after use, many doctors feel they are prescribed much too often and for over too long a period of time for many patients. Before these drugs came along, phenobarbital and chloral hydrate were the drugs of choice for treating anxiety, and it is still not convincingly shown that the new drugs are any more effective. Phenobarbital and chloral hydrate are certainly less expensive, in some cases one-tenth the cost of the meprobamates.

One problem with the antihistamines, when used for treating hay fever, is the drowsiness they cause. This is a distinct liability for the hay fever patient but an asset if people want to go to sleep. It naturally followed that the drug could serve as a switch-hitter, and the over-the-counter sales of antihistamines as sleeping pills have proved to be a commercial success. Dr. Hollister warns, however, that this kind of use has never been properly examined. He discourages use of antihistamines as sedatives because they are not very effective and are "quite toxic" in overdoses.

Dr. Hollister, who has assembled and organized massive information on this entire psychotropic field of drugs, feels that patients with anxiety symptoms should first be given phenobarbitol and then *if necessary* be moved to the meprobamates.

Hypnotics make up the class commonly known as sleeping pills and, again, are widely overprescribed. Insomnia haunts a large percentage of the population. Most expert opinion is that they should be used sparingly and intermittently. There's no question that they do induce sleep, but anyone who has taken them knows the sluggish type of hangover that results. Further, a series of very interesting dream studies has shown that the sleeping pill-hypnotic drugs cause severe "dream deprivation," which is suspected to have serious effects on the psyche.

The hypnotics are close cousins to the antianxiety and sedative drugs and often "may be interchangeable according to the dosage used." Chloral hydrate seems to interfere with normal sleep the least. Authorities state that its use as the "Mickey Finn" of barroom fame is largely a myth. A phenobarbital substitute known as glutethimide (Doriden) might be effective in bringing about a drugged sleep. However, a warning is out that it is highly dangerous both for potential abuse and for serious problems connected with any overdose. The Federal Supply Agency won't buy it anymore.

So-called *skeletal muscle relaxants* have come into great popularity, especially for things like a stiff neck or back strain. They are often combined with aspirin or aspirin compounds, and the National Institutes of Health attributes a lot of their pain-killing qualities to this. Again, these are close chemical cousins to the meprobomates, are basically sedatives, and most probably are no better than meprobamate or phenobarbital and a hot bath for dealing with this sort of situation.

Analgesics are not really part of the psychotropic scene but are often classified with them. But, as Dr. Hollister says: "Aspirin is one of the wonder drugs of all time. Correctly used, it can afford relief for many discomforts, often being adequate for degrees of pain thought to require more potent drugs. Aspirin compound (aspirin, phenacetin, and caffeine, known as APC), although widely used, is no better than aspirin and may not be as good, for phenacetin is not as effective an analgesic as aspirin. [If you buy aspirin, buy the "house" brand. It is no different from Bayer and often costs less than half as much.] Codeine is a different type of drug, being related to morphine. It is well absorbed by mouth (other opiates are not), more analgesic than aspirin but less so than morphine, and safe in the usual doses."

All drugs are dangerous, of course, but aspirin is deceivingly so because it is so widely used. One doctor in Connecticut said that he was most distressed by the constant number of cases coming into the emergency room of his hospital with internal bleeding resulting from aspirin. In spite of its great benefits, aspirin is dangerous and should always be used with caution. Rare deaths have occurred even through light to moderate usage. Some recommend a full glass of milk with aspirin in order to retard the serious internal burns it can cause at times. Other doctors recommend taking sodium bicarbonate tablets with the aspirin or half a teaspoon of baking soda in water. If a real aspirin allergy exists, acetaminophen is often used as a substitute.

The search for a better analgesic than aspirin is continually going on, but the progress is not good. Parke, Davis tried with a product they called Ponstel (mefanamic acid). With the usual misled vigor, it began to push the drug onto the medical profession, touting it as a super pain killer and playing down the fact that the drug should never be taken longer than a week at most. The company plugged the results of a highly inadequate clinical test, without bothering to include several other tests. Some of them showed that aspirin was actually better than the expensive brand name Ponstel, which fared in the tests exactly the same as a dummy medication placebo.

By far the most controversial of the analgesics is Darvon, known generically as propoxyphene. There are some facts that the layman should know about this drug. First, in pharmacologically equivalent doses, it is not one whit better than aspirin. Some studies show it to be inferior. Second, it costs forty to fifty times as much. Third, it has a distinct family resemblance to its siblings, codeine, morphine, heroin, and methadone. It is closest to methadone, which is the drug used to replace heroin in addiction withdrawal. Fourth, Darvon's use can result in acute withdrawal symptoms, including convulsions and coma. Fifth, it is the most overprescribed drug in the country—more prescriptions are dispensed in retail pharmacies for Darvon than for any other drug, according to the American Medical Association. In comparing Darvon to aspirin or APC, the authoritative *Medical Letter* says that Darvon ". . . has consistently proven inferior to aspirin or APC tablets. No evidence that has appeared since this review [of recent studies] has established the superiority of the 65 milligram doses of propoxyphene (Darvon) to two tablets of either aspirin or APC."

According to the most expert testimony available, that is the story on Darvon. This evidence is thought to be incontestable. Why it continues to be prescribed at this overwhelming rate is anybody's guess, but the manufacturer does not seem to be bothering to check the drift.

Stimulants, according to Dr. Hollister's careful and comprehensive analysis, are dominated by the amphetamines (more technically, dextroamphetamines), and when they were introduced over three decades ago, there was nothing better to pep up the sluggish, eliminate that tired feeling, and bring about a roseate haze of euphoria.

The problem, of course, is that the amphetamines have become a major scene on the drug abuse front, to say nothing of their overuse in prescription traffic and for diet control as appetite depressants.

Even the most hardened drug abuser is wary of the amphetamines because he knows they are killers. "Speed kills" is the byword of the drug scene, and it is no idle phrase. When they are taken orally, the drug user calls them speed. When they are taken intravenously, they are known as crystal. Crashing from speed or crystal is the most agonizing, horrifying experience encountered in drug abuse. A speed freak is the saddest of all drug trippers.

The mass production of amphetamines goes far beyond the logical, clinical use of the drug. In late 1971, the Department of Justice cut the quotas for the production of amphetamines by 40 percent, a long-delayed necessity in combating drug abuse. Since many experts feel that at least 50 percent of these drugs have been going into illicit drug traffic, those who are fighting for drug control feel that the government action is too little and too late. The pharmaceutical industry, of course, protested loudly because it had demanded 70 percent more production than the new quota permitted. 1972 is the first year the government has been able to set production quotas for these dangerous drugs.

Just how many amphetamine tablets find their way to Mexico and abroad and then return by illegal channels is hard to pin down. There is serious concern that the pharmaceutical companies are producing far too much of the amphetamine product for any sensible use via legitimate prescription channels. A recent article in the prestigious *Annals of Internal Medicine* states that 99 percent of all production is superfluous. Just what the drug companies are doing to prevent this export-import gambit is not discernible. But the attitude of the Pharmaceutical Manufacturers Association borders on criminal indifference.

In a report to Senator Gaylord Nelson, this association attempted to point up the basic reasons why the drug companies required such high profits (even though profits are not at all required to pay for research, which is a cost-of-goods-sold item). One of its complaints was that the manufacturer faces sharp financial loss when one or more of its standby drugs becomes an object of drug abuse. Without alluding to the possibility that if a manufacturer is not aware of one of its drugs being abused it must be blind as a bat, the PMA report says:

> The most dangerous drugs have been withdrawn from the market or not permitted to be marketed in the first place. Other drugs, addictive derivatives of opium, have been placed under the strict controls of the Narcotics Bureau. But there is an important third category of drugs, including the barbiturates and the amphetamines, which are of proven value and far less dangerous, which have been found only recently to be subject to abuse and have hence been made subject to the Drug Abuse Control Act.
>
> The removal of a product from non-prescription status, or if already a legend drug, the placing of that product under the restrictions of the Drug Abuse Control Act *is likely to have a depressing effect on sales* and as such must be considered as one of the risks facing the industry. [The italics are the author's.]

Only one thing is on the mind of this fantastic and unbelievably archaic organization—*a depressing effect on sales.* Not one word about the speed freaks, about the illicit traffic in the "ethically produced" drugs, not one word of concern about how to stop it, not one thought apparently about why there was so much production of barbiturates and amphetamines to begin with, not one word about the plush, lush, lavish ads in the medical journals, brainwashing doctors to overprescribe these escape pellets from the realities and normal stresses of life.

The Pharmaceutical Manufacturers Association goes on to say: "Smith, Kline and French has estimated the loss of sales on its amphetamine products due to the new Drug Abuse Control Act restrictions at about 20 per cent for this important category of its product line."

Obviously, if the sales have dropped 20 percent because of the new drug abuse restrictions, this means that 20 percent of its giant "speed" production has been going into illegal channels all along—or else *why* would it drop? And if this 20 percent of production was getting into the wrong hands, why didn't the company know it—and stop it? Certainly it must have been obvious to SKF executives that the extra production must have exceeded the legitimate prescription trade. Or if not, why not? And with extra profits coming from illegal traffic, how could any socially conscious executive in his right mind lament giving them up under such circumstances? And how would the Pharmaceutical Manufacturers Association garner the unmitigated gall to present this as an argument, deadpan and serious? The words were actually written down on paper and were sent to Senator Nelson with an accompanying letter signed by C. Joseph Stetler on the Pharmaceutical Manufacturers Association letterhead, and Mr. Stetler is the certified chief executive of that organization.

The PMA's continuous and unrelenting fight to prevent the doctor from prescribing by generic name of the drug instead of the brand name is just another part of this profits-first, people-last attitude in the psychotropic drugs as in all the others. Its member companies will go to great lengths in order to make it almost impossible for a doctor to prescribe anything but the original brand name. An example is Darvon. Henry Steele, of Rice University, reports in an article for the *Journal of Law and Economics* that drug makers are free to designate the generic name for any new compound they put on the market. They take considerable pains to make sure that the generic name will be about as difficult as it can be for the doctor to remember and, by the same token, make sure that the brand name is simple and easy to remember.*

In the case of Darvon, the makers anointed it with the generic name of *dextropropohyphene hydrochloride.*

Which is the name the doctor will write on the prescription blank?

* Dr. Richard Burack is actively trying to fight this practice. He is chairman of the Massachusetts Drug Formulary Commission, whose job is to administer a prototype law making it mandatory for Massachusetts doctors to put generic names on prescription blanks. His commission has compiled and distributed to every doctor in the state an educational list of generic and brand equivalent names. The PMA hates him. Among doctors he's their public enemy number one whose name and book (*The New Handbook of Prescription Drugs*) are never to be mentioned. But the new generation of medical students look to Burack as a hero.

7

The Bigger the Stranger, the Softer the Bark

OVER a period of fifteen years, Dr. Paul Lowinger, associate professor of psychiatry at Wayne State University medical school and also chief of the outpatient service of the Lafayette Clinic in Detroit, worked on the development and evaluation of many of the new drugs that skyrocketed into broad use during that time. He felt part of the new tide that resulted in such popularity for these drugs was the fact that they were instrumental in bringing about such a revolution in the care of the mentally ill, so that many could be released from hospitals who had no hope before.

But he was also concerned about the health and safety of the patients receiving the new medications. He was assured by the pharmaceutical companies for whom he conducted controlled clinical tests that his results would be carefully reported to the FDA, so that an objective appraisal of a new drug could be made before it was permitted to go on the market. In all, he conducted some twenty-seven new drug studies.

"The seeds of doubt began in 1965," he told Senator Nelson's subcommittee, "when I learned that our findings on the safety of Dornwal, studied in 1961 for Wallace and Tiernan (the manufacturer of the drug), had not been reported to the Food and Drug Administration. The reason for the eventual government prosecution of Wallace & Tiernan was that serious and fatal toxic effects of Dornwal on the blood had not been reported to the FDA."

With rather sluggish cooperation from the FDA, he discovered in his own studies that only nine of the twenty-seven drug studies he had conducted had been submitted to the FDA. The others were covered up. Some of the adverse reactions which the companies had failed to pass along in their new drug applications included dizziness, drowsiness, mood depression, anxiety, insomnia, blurred vision, loss of anal sphincter control, ringing in the ears, headaches, itching dermatitis, weakness, fatigue, nausea, diarrhea, abdominal distress, constipation, and a possible case of hepatitis.

The Dornwal cover-up was more profound. Its use brought on serious blood dyscrasias, uncovered by the same Dr. Frances Kelsey who had spiked the wide use of thalidomide in this country.

The willful concealing of adverse reaction reports seems to be widespread among both the smaller and the larger manufacturers. McNeil Laboratories, Inc., a subsidiary of Johnson & Johnson, was accused by HEW of covering up over a two-year period very serious side reactions to its drug Flexin, which allegedly caused serious liver damage, anemia, and leukopenia, among other effects. According to HEW, between August, 1956, and October, 1958, McNeil Laboratories received reports of twenty-six cases of liver damage in Flexin patients of whom seven died. Allegedly, false and misleading statements were constantly made by the company in its attempt to keep the drug on the market. The Department of Justice refused to prosecute because the action was barred by the statute of limitations and because supplemental drug applications submitted by McNeil sufficiently disclosed the possibility of liver damage.

This habitual practice of trying to cover up the damage drugs can do to patients and the failure to provide adequate warnings to the doctor has led to an endless parade of "Dear Doctor" letters, which the FDA forces the pharmaceutical companies to send out, under the pain of glaring bad publicity about their products. The companies fight against this letter of apology, knowing that every "Dear Doctor" letter they are forced to send out means loss of sales. The fact that such a letter might save the lives of some of the patients taking their drugs does not seem to figure in the scheme of things.

Over an eighteen-month period, twenty-nine "Dear Doctor" letters were required to be sent out by many of the leading companies in the trade. They included: Hoffman-LaRoche for Librium; Wallace Laboratories for Deprol and Miltown; Abbott Laboratories for Enduron, Enduronyl, and Erythrocin; Parke, Davis for Ponstel; Mead-Johnson for Oracon and Questran; Pfizer for Rondomycin and others; Squibb for Mysteclin-F; Upjohn for Medrol; Bristol for Dynapen; Warner-Chilcott for Nebair; Schick Safety Razor (pharmaceutical division) for Enzopride; Dupont for Symmetrel; and CIBA for Ismelin.

In the letters, the companies do everything they can to soft-pedal the bad news the FDA makes them send along to the doctors. Typical phrases in the letters run something like this one that Roche Laboratories sent out in regard to Librium:

> The statement that "Side effects in most instances are mild in degree and readily reversible with reduction of dosage" will be extended by the observations made in our package circular which point out that drowsiness, ataxia [loss of muscular coordination], and confusion have been reported in some patients, particularly the elderly and debilitated, occasionally at lower dosage ranges, and that in a few instances, syncope [loss of consciousness from transient hypotension] has been reported.

The FDA does not require the companies to explain just why they left out warnings of this kind in the first place. In this case, the warning was already in the package insert, which the physician rarely reads. It is an interesting speculation why Roche left it out of the medical journal advertisement, which the doctor is more likely to read.

In other "Dear Doctor" letters, Mead-Johnson was forced to spell out the following about its Oracon contraceptive:

It [the medical journal ad] fails to give adequate emphasis to
more serious known side effects—or adequate emphasis to the
possible occurrence of thrombophlebitis, pulmonary embolism
or cerebral vascular accident.

Warner-Chilcott was forced to include in its letter to the
doctors certain side effects it conveniently forgot to list regarding its aerosol inhalator Nebair. They included: vomiting, headaches, flushing of the skin, tremor, weakness,
sweating, and angina-type pain. It also neglected to remind
the doctor that frequent or continuous use on a long-term
basis is not recommended and that use in children under
twelve is not indicated. These are things that would be nice
for a doctor to be able to tell a patient, in case any of the
symptoms sprang up unexpectedly.

When Commissioner Charles Edwards stepped into his job
as head of the FDA, he not only inherited this problem, but
many others as well. It is doubtful if anyone envies his responsibilities, although it is certain that many admire his
daring. His background is steeped in medicine—as a physician, surgeon, and teacher of medicine, including Princeton,
University of Colorado, Minnesota, the Mayo Clinic, and
other distinguished institutions. He has the further periph-
eral asset of being strikingly handsome, with a distinguished
crop of premature gray hair that prompts a generous handful
of FDA secretaries to keep his picture on the wall near their
desks. In addition to that, he has shown very clear evidence
of being alert, perceptive, quick to grasp essential facts and to
drive swiftly to the heart of the problem.

What has not shown up clearly is his basic attitude toward
the food, drug, and cosmetic industries, for which he is the
appointed watchdog. Among myriads of other problems,
some of the first things on Commissioner Edwards' mind as
he took over the key to his office included several specific
problems in the prescription drug field.

The hottest item at the time was the oral contraceptive situation. For perhaps the first time in history, perfectly healthy
people, millions of them, were on a regular regimen of phar-

maceutical prescription drugs. Commissioner Edwards had already been raked by Senator Nelson's Senate Monopoly Subcommittee in early spring on the subject; his baptism was comparatively gentle.

One of the reasons for Senator Nelson's uncharacteristic soft touch was Commissioner Edwards' disarming frankness in admitting the new dangers that were then arising about "the Pill" and his firm resolve to take an unprecedented step: to require a 600-word warning package insert that each patient would have to receive with her package of tablets.

Senator Nelson commended Edwards highly for his initiative in the service of the patient, and Edwards went into detail about how the warning leaflet would explain to the patient that there is a risk of blood clotting for pill users that is six times higher than for nonusers. The areas most likely for this would be in the legs, lungs, or brain. The proposed statement for the package insert also warned against the use of the pill by those who had liver disease, cancer of the breast, heart or kidney disease, asthma, high blood pressure, diabetes, epilepsy, fibroids of the uterus, migraine headaches, or mental depression. It also warned of the possibility of the pill creating swelling, skin rash, jaundice, increase in blood pressure or blood sugar level, nervousness, dizziness, and several other reactions that the pill had been known to cause in certain instances. The proposed warning ended with a note about cancer: "Scientists know the hormones in the pill (estrogen and progesterone) have caused cancer in animals, but they have no proof that the pill causes cancer in humans. Because your doctor knows this, he will want to examine you regularly."

The Nelson committee was also pleased with the frankness of the new FDA approach when it was admitted that changes in the labeling of the pill met with considerable resistance from the pharmaceutical industry. Summarizing his feelings about Commissioner Edwards' attitude, Senator Nelson said:

"I do want to say Commissioner Edwards, who has only been in office for a few months, has moved vigorously in this area and has taken an historic action that no previous Commissioner before has ever taken, that it certainly required courage to do so, because I am familiar with the medical politics involved."

And there *were* politics involved—plenty of them. They began moving with fury after Edwards' appearance before the Nelson committee. The drug companies, along with the American Medical Association, immediately closed in on Edwards' gallant statement. Very shortly after, and without ceremony, Edwards cut the 600-word stern warning down to 96 words, much milder. Instead of including a specific list of dangers, the new statement pointed only to one. It also did not include instructions as to when a woman taking the pill should see her doctor. Senator Nelson's admiration was short-lived.

Apparently, immediately after Edwards had announced his plans at the Senate hearing, the AMA put pressure on Dr. Roger Egeberg, Assistant HEW Secretary, as well as HEW Secretary Finch. The motive was supposedly the jealous guarding of doctor-patient relationships. The drug companies objected strenuously that the 600-word statement overemphasized the dangers. It was reported that Edwards was in the doghouse for announcing the plan without letting the top HEW brass know ahead of time. Egeberg is supposed to have pressured Edwards into slashing the warning down to its more innocuous form. One Senator told a New York *Times* reporter his reaction to the microversion of the warning: "Any similarity between this draft and what the FDA proposed [at the Nelson hearings] is purely coincidental."

Senator Thomas McIntyre, of the Nelson committee, was considerably upset. "I am deeply disturbed by the press stories indicating that the Food and Drug Administration has watered down the consumer labeling for birth control pills."

So intense was the reaction in some quarters that two members of the Women's Liberation Movement stormed the FDA bastille to crash in on an Advisory Committee meeting there to demand that the full warning be reinstated.

Edwards tried to explain the whole thing away by saying:

"The more we got to thinking about it, the more we thought that we had put too much clinical material in it." He added that he had two objectives: to warn the 8,500,000 pill users that the pill is a safe but potent drug, and to remind doctors to follow up patients taking the drug very closely.

Edwards, who has insisted all along that he would not have taken the Commissioner's job unless he would have the freedom to make his own decisions, denied that he had been pressured into watering down the warning by his bosses in the HEW.

Yet it was HEW Secretary Finch, not Commissioner Edwards, who announced the short-form draft of the warning on April 7, 1970. It had been extended now to 120 words, still nearly 500 words short of the version presented to the Senate committee. It included five symptoms to look for that the 96-word version had left out: (1) severe headache, (2) blurred vision, (3) pain in the legs, (4) pain in the chest or unexplained cough, and (5) irregular or missed periods. In spite of these additions, it was still weaker than the original proposed by Edwards.

Senator Nelson was not too happy about it. A *Newsweek* poll had shown that two out of every three women taking the pill had not been warned at all by their doctors. The Senator indicated that one of the sentences in the new Finch-announced warning that bothered him was: "Rare instances of abnormal blood clotting are the most important known complication of the oral contraceptives."

"In my own subjective judgment," the Senator said, "the word 'rare' is inaccurate as used here, since the hospitalization rates due to thrombo-embolic ["thrombo" refers to a clot, "embolism" to a piece that breaks off from the clot] is one in two thousand."

One of the strongest protesters against the 600-word warning when it was announced was G. D. Searle & Company, makers of oral contraceptive Enovid. This company's stance, along with other makers and the AMA, which promised a legal battle against the warning, were directly challenging a critical issue: the public's right to know. Searle's Enovid had been the issue in the case of Elizabeth Black, who died at the age of twenty-nine from a pulmonary embolism. Particles of the clot were found in the veins leading from the ovaries to the lungs. These were typical symptoms that were gathering statistically in the users of Enovid, and they were alarming. The Searle company was stalling on new studies to check this out, even though several expert medical committees had recommended them.

When Elizabeth Black died, her widower brought an unsuccessful suit against Searle to collect damages, but expert testimony at the trial revealed that the company was continuing to avoid any clear and concise warning about the dangers of the pill. In a cross-examination at the trial, Dr. Irwin Winter, of Searle, was questioned about the pamphlet Searle provided the doctors to give to their patients. The plaintiff's attorney questioned Dr. Winter in detail about this:

Q. . . . . the company knew that when these [the Searle pamphlets] were given to the patient the patient would rely on them in the use of the pill?
A. As far as the booklets went, yes.
Q. Now, there's nothing in these booklets, Doctor, that talked about what to do if they had any chest pains, was there?
A. No, sir.
Q. Or what to do if they suddenly started breaking out in a sweat with chest pain?
A. No.
Q. Or other symptoms that have to do with an embolism, is there?
A. No.
Q. Or shortness of breath?
A. No, sir.
Q. You talk about morning sickness, don't you?
A. Right.
Q. That's not fatal, is it?
A. Not usually. . . .
Q. Yes. Well, in this booklet, you say some people experience weight gain?
A. That's right.

Q. Right. Some people experience thrombo-embolisms, too, don't they?
A. We know that happens, yes. They experience a lot of other things, too, though.
Q. Doctor, why is it that you didn't put in these booklets the warnings about this potentially deadly thrombo-embolism?

Dr. Winter tried to explain that to do that would require giving a woman a full course in medicine. This seemed hardly an adequate explanation in the face of the 400-plus incidents of clotting among the users of Enovid.

The problem of the pill is acute and perplexing in the face of the fact that population control is one of the most important issues of the day. Senator Nelson, a great supporter of population control, was driving only at the irresponsibility of the drug companies in not forewarning the public and the doctors about the dangers. He was not against the pill itself. As in all the excesses of the pharmaceutical firms, the sales, advertising, and promotion efforts were the heavy villain, constantly covering up bad news and exaggerating good news. In no other field is this control so vital and important.

By the time the controversy generated by the Nelson Senate committee had simmered down, a new explosion flared up: The warning statement that HEW Secretary Finch had announced, and which was officially printed in the *Federal Register*, had been *again* chopped down to remove *any* mention of the specific symptoms the patient was to watch out for. It was at this point that Congressman Fountain's House Intergovernmental Relations Subcommittee stepped in to press Edwards on the reason for this obvious concession to pharmaceutical industry pressure. Edwards tried to explain this away with some strange, wandering language that sounded for all the world like double talk. He contended that the FDA should "go all the way or none at all in terms of listing symptoms," whatever that means. He said that "looking at seven and only seven symptoms really did not give the user the information that she should have"—whatever that means. He tried to explain that the doctor was supposed to pass this information along to the patient, but he did not explain why, if the patient was going to get this warning from the doctor, she shouldn't have a reminder of it in the package insert. Again, the public's right to know was at stake.

The new and weakened warning did include a statement to the effect that a booklet telling the patient about the effectiveness and hazards of the pill would be available from the doctor on request. This, Edwards indicated, would be cleared through the FDA. If the wording of this booklet were to be anything like the original package inserts of the pill makers, it would again reflect the consummate skill of the advertising copy man's euphemisms. For instance, one of the earlier "instructional" pieces read:

> So close to your natural feminine pattern. Your doctor has prescribed this newest kind of fertility-control tablet for you. Unlike others available for the same purpose, this preparation follows the principle and system of nature itself. Its actions closely resemble those of your natural menstrual pattern, and it works without upsetting the delicate balance of your normal body functions.

That this is utter balderdash, that it ignores serious side effects and reactions, that it assures safety when safety cannot be assured never seems to enter the manufacturer's mind.

More specifically, Congressman Fountain's subcommittee was interested in another oral contraceptive of G. D. Searle & Company, a newer one called Demulen. Supposedly this drug was to follow the discoveries in England that the lower-level estrogen compounds were just as effective as the higher-level pills and reduced the overexposure of the system to estrogen. Actually, the clinical studies for Demulen showed no reduction in side effects compared to other common oral contraceptives. Some tests that were purported to prove this were judged useless. The Searle new drug application for Demulen was passed by the FDA, because it was at least no worse than others on the market.

However, when it came to advertising the product Searle outdid itself. The medical journal advertising stated that Demulen "offers added assurance in view of today's concern." Called on the carpet again by the Fountain subcommittee, Commissioner Edwards frankly admitted that the Demulen ad was obviously false.

Then Congressman Fountain asked him: "Do you have in mind taking any action with respect to this particular advertisement which you said was misleading?"

"Mr. Chairman," Commissioner Edwards replied, "to the best of my knowledge we have had no official communications with the Searle Company. I might ask Dr. Simmons if they have any immediate plans. This is the Division of Drug Advertising."

Dr. Henry Simmons, head of the FDA's Bureau of Drugs, replied: "First of all, I'm not sure that the statement by the Commissioner really said that."

"He said it," Fountain replied. "Later he may have modified it."

"There is no doubt it is a safe and effective compound," Dr. Simmons continued. "It just doesn't have less side effects than another thing. It is equally protective against contraception. That is true in the ad. The fact that it may be better than others, which is inferred, is what we object to and plan to inform the firm about."

Fountain answered: "I notice you keep using the term 'safe and effective.' That is not at issue. We are not raising questions about safety and efficacy."

"It becomes an issue," said Dr. Simmons, "only because the ad for this product infers [he meant "implies" in both cases] that it may be even better in effectiveness than another. This we can't say for sure. We know it is a low dose estrogen and hope that will make a difference. But to say in a definite statement that this is superior to, we object to that. All the contraceptives are safe and effective and have about the same side effects. That is what we object to in the tone."

Referring to the Searle ad, Fountain said: "This goes beyond that. It says: 'Announcing the half-new pill.'"

Dr. Edwards broke into the duologue to say: "That too is misleading."

Congressman Fountain's patience was wearing thin. "That is an outright lie, isn't it?" he snapped.

When Simmons tried to explain that he didn't seem to get that inference, staff professional D. C. Goldberg cut in on the conversation. "Drug advertising is a very specialized field, Dr. Simmons," he said to the newly appointed bureau head. "I don't know whether you have any expertise in it or not."

Then after asking whether Dr. Simmons had checked with his drug advertising department, Dr. Goldberg continued: "You know all about this drug. The purpose of the advertising is to convey the impression that the manufacturer has a superior product, as well as to pass on information. The average physician, unless he has studied the record of how Demulen was approved, and is aware of the kind of evidence that was presented for the drug's effectiveness and safety, cannot judge whether or not the ad is misleading. That is the job of the FDA, to decide whether or not the ad was misleading.

"I talked to two physicians in the last two days and they were horrified. They thought this was a terrible misleading ad. If physicians can come away with differing impressions of the facts an advertisement is intended to convey, that is a very undesirable situation. What we are looking for is truth in advertising; that is what the advertising provisions of the Food and Drug Act are all about."

Whatever Dr. Simmons thought about the situation—he seemed a little naïve and confused about the subtleties of the drug advertisers—he whisked a letter off to Searle on July 20, 1970, three days after the hearing, requiring that the schedule for the ad be canceled. Searle replied that they did not agree at all that the ad was misleading but reluctantly agreed to suspend publication of the ads.

It is little wonder that the users of the pill were totally confused by this time. In an effort to make their oral contraceptives a surefire barrier against pregnancy, many manufacturers were loading their pills with .075 milligrams, or more, of estrogen, when .05 milligrams was sufficient to prevent conception. It took news from the British Committee on Safety of Drugs to point this out and to advise physicians in England to prescribe the lower dose. The British studies showed there was far less blood clotting resulting from the weaker product. In the beginning of 1970, Edwards failed to take the same action as the British committee did but merely recommended to doctors that they make patients "fully aware of the risks involved." He indicated new FDA studies would be conducted.

At about the same time, January, 1970, the *Congressional Quarterly* summed up the testimony of several doctors before the Nelson committee.

From Dr. Hugh J. Davis, director of the Contraceptive Clinic at Johns Hopkins:

> Birth control pills might cause breast cancer that would not be detected for years. The same synthetic hormones in the pill have induced breast cancer in five different species of animals. Every important agent which has a carcinogenic (cancer-producing) effect in humans has been shown to cause cancer in animals.
>
> Physical examinations would not necessarily protect women against metabolic changes or breast cancer that might be caused by the pill because of the difficulties in detecting such changes. By the time the doctor found a lump, the cancer could have been there for years.
>
> Other contraceptive devices and methods are almost as effective as the pill and much safer. . . .

From Dr. Roy Hertz, of Rockefeller University's Population Council:

> Only two things have been substantiated about The Pill: Its high degree of effectiveness in preventing pregnancy, and its ability to cause blood clotting. Estrogens are to breast cancer what fertilizer is to the wheat crop.

From Dr. Edmond Kassouf, an internist from Cranford, New Jersey:

Drug companies try to suppress reports about dangers in the use of the pill. Known hazards are denied and distorted in the literature put out by the companies. Major concerns are casually treated or ignored. Some of the pamphlets mislead and misinform. Others are frankly dangerous.

From Dr. Marvin Legator, the outspoken FDA chief of cell biology:

The earliest period for detecting an increase in breast cancer among women who started using the pill in the early 1960's, would be in the 1970's because the disease lies dormant for many years. The only data which scientists have on the effects of the pill came from animal testing. Further testing is needed on the possibility of mutations resulting from widespread use of the pill.

Even though Commissioner Edwards knew about the British studies in January, it took until April 24, 1970, for the FDA to come out with a press release recommending flatly that doctors prescribe those pills that contain the lowest amount of estrogen. Up until this time, only about half of the 8,500,000 users were on the lower .05-milligram dose. In other words, some 4,000,000 women had been regularly using from .06- to .10-milligram dosages, pills that were producing two to three times the number of blood-clotting experiences. Among these obviously dangerous powerhouse pills were: Enovid, C-Quens, Ovulen, and Oracon. Some American brands under the .05-milligram limit of safety are Ortho-Novum, Norinyl, and Norlestrin.

Whether it was a coincidence or not, the publication of the press release announcing the package insert to be required of all oral contraceptive manufacturers took place on June 9, 1970, the day that Commissioner Edwards was called up before Congressman Fountain's House committee to report on many things, including the Pill.

The package insert, a hash concocted by the fine hands of Finch, Egeberg, the AMA, the PMA, and Edwards, finally read as follows:

ORAL CONTRACEPTIVES
(Birth Control Pills)

> Do not take this drug without your
> Doctor's continued supervision.

Oral contraceptives are powerful and effective drugs which can cause side effects in some users and should not be used at all by some women. The most serious known side effect is abnormal blood clotting which can be fatal.

Safe use of this drug requires a careful discussion with your doctor. To assist him in providing you with the necessary information, (Firm name) has prepared a booklet (or other form) written in a style understandable to you as the drug user. This provides comprehensive information on the effectiveness and known hazards of the drug including warnings, side effects and who should not use it. Your doctor will give you this booklet (or other form) and answer any questions you may have about the use of this drug.

Notify your doctor if you notice any unusual physical disturbances or discomfort.

By August, 1970, Commissioner Edwards had worked out the copy for the longer, more comprehensive booklet with the cooperation of the American Medical Association. Edwards was happy about the whole thing, stating that the cooperative job was "a good example of how the public and private sectors can work together" despite the "differences of opinion involved."

Dr. Max Parrott, chairman of the AMA board of trustees, announced that the main goal was to assure that each patient taking the pill is seeing a physician. "There's only one person," he told the *American Medical News*, "who can judge if the pill is safe for an individual. And that's your physician— not your Senator."

The last crack was an obvious swipe at Senator Gaylord Nelson and his committee.

An interesting sidelight on the development of the booklet was that the Pharmaceutical Manufacturers Association slapped at the AMA-FDA co-op effort, contending that more recent studies on the risks of the pill were not as great as the AMA pamphlet indicated. The AMA figures showed that the chances of blood clotting in healthy women under thirty-five is over six times greater for those who take the pill than for those who don't. Question: Which do you believe—the American Medical Association (in this case at least) or the Pharmaceutical Manufacturers Association?

By October, 1970, some of the drug makers began to get the message. Eli Lilly and Upjohn "voluntarily" stopped the manufacture of their two high-potency estrogen pills, C-Quens and Provest, respectively. It had been discovered that beagle dogs given ten to twenty-five times the human dose developed breast nodules at an earlier age and in larger numbers than did control dogs not given the drug. The findings had not been reproduced in dogs that had received other oral contraceptives. At this stage, the nodules had shown no malignancy. At the conclusion of the FDA press release, Commissioner Edwards emphasized there was no cause for patient alarm and that women taking either C-Quens or Provest should continue until advised by their physicians on a change.

With this, one chapter of the history of the Pill had come to an end. Where it would go next, few, if any, could predict. It took twenty years for the problem of estrogen and cervical cancer in the new generation to show up.

If the theory is valid that the promotion and advertising of a drug can be as hazardous to the eventual consumer as the drug itself, Commissioner Edwards had plenty to worry about the minute he took up his duties, and Congressman Fountain's House committee was not going to let him forget. He was reminded at a hearing that some very specific cases of FDA sluggishness in moving against the drug companies needed some explanation, if not from Edwards, from Dr. Simmons, his drug bureau head.

In one case, U.S. Vitamin ran a misleading ad on its oral diabetic drug DBI-TD in December, 1969. The FDA wrote the company shortly after, and it agreed to stop the ad. Three months later, another objectionable ad appeared. The FDA medical staff recommended to Dr. Simmons that another warning letter be sent. It wasn't. Three months later, in June, another misleading ad appeared.

In an attempt to explain this beneficent tolerance for a company that was repeatedly violating FDA directives, Dr. Edwards told the hearing: "As you know there has been a recent study by a group in regard to oral anti-diabetics, and this created a tremendous amount of controversy in the medical field. We are at the moment working with the American Diabetic Association, with other scientific medical groups . . . At an appropriate time, we will be sending a communication to doctors.

"I do not think this necessarily excuses our allowing this advertisement to continue, but I think it does indicate that we have at least rationalized it in terms of trying to deal with the bigger problem."

Congressman Fountain replied: "I do not understand that attitude. That is like saying we have a law on the books against a serious violation, but because the law is going to be changed sometime soon we are not going to do anything against the violators of existing law. . . .

"Dr. Edwards, don't you agree that if the firm promotes the drug through misleading advertising on a national scale, action should be taken regardless of the state of labeling revision under consideration?"

"Absolutely," Dr. Edwards replied.

"Then what do you plan to do about this advertisement?" Congressman Fountain asked.

"It will be corrected as of possibly even today," said Edwards, as the hearing room rippled with a wave of laughter.

There was no question about it; the oral diabetic drugs were having almost as rough a time as the oral contraceptives. The FDA was at this point taking action against Upjohn's Orinase (tolbutamide), which not only appeared to be no more effective than diet alone but showed significantly that more people who took Orinase were dying than those control groups who were not taking the drug.

During approximately the same time period, the large and powerful corporation of Smith Kline & French came out with an ad bristling with misinformation for its drug Dyrenium. This drug's usefulness was limited to the treatment of certain kinds of edema, which is an excessive accumulation of fluid in the tissues. In other words, it is a very special kind of diuretic drug, those designed to increase the production of urine. Although the general class of diuretics is also used in the treatment of hypertension, Dyrenium was not indicated for this purpose.

Especially interesting was that this advertisement was drawn up in cooperation with the highly regarded *New England Journal of Medicine*, which was claiming to seek ways to put a stop to all the continual abuses the drug companies were subjecting their doctor readers to in the professional journals. In fact, the *New England Journal* came out with a glowing editorial about the Dyrenium ad, lavishly praising Smith Kline & French's taste and recognition of precautions to be taken with the use of the drug. The drug trade press joined in the chorus of approval of this perfect "model ad" that would certainly win all the awards in that big pharmaceutical record book in the sky.

But when the ad came out, the medical experts at the FDA found a few problems with it. Smith Kline & French neglected to mention to doctor readers that Dyrenium was approved *only* for the treatment of edema, and that only from certain specific causes. It further neglected to point out that the drug was to be used as a diuretic only for the above causes. With these omissions, the ad implied that it was safe and effective for all conditions treatable by any other diuretic, including hypertension. Because of this, a physician might well be conned into prescribing it for a hypertensive patient, when Dyrenium had never been established for such use. The ad further implied it was more economical than all other diuretics, which was grossly misleading.

The reaction of FDA's H. W. Chadduck, acting director of the Division of Drug Advertising, was sharp and trenchant. "This is perhaps one of the most important ad cases the FDA has had," he wrote to his department chief.

"As background, Smith Kline & French Laboratories has

some regulatory history on advertising matters. The firm has been warned at least three times on violations (Thorazine, 1964; Dexamyl Spansules, 1966; Eskatrol, 1969). The firm has not issued a remedial letter in the past, but has acknowledged errors by changing a specific advertising practice when warned about it. The immediate situation outlined above is regarded as serious, and comparable with those in the past which have resulted in seizures, prosecutions, and 'Dear Doctor' letters."

The violative ad appeared in February, 1970. By mid-July, no corrective ads had been published. During this time, behind the scenes at the FDA strange things were happening. When the clarion call for obvious direct and immediate action reached the desk of Dr. Henry Simmons, Director of the Bureau of Drugs for the FDA, the shrill tones of the trumpet apparently did not reach his ear. For instance, Commissioner Edwards' letter to Smith Kline & French insisted that the company run a remedial ad with a box reading: PUBLISHED TO REPLACE A PREVIOUS ADVERTISEMENT WHICH THE FOOD AND DRUG ADMINISTRATION CONSIDERED MISLEADING.

The situation dealt with a large corporation and with a prestigious medical journal that had beat the drums for the "model ad." Strangely enough, Smith Kline & French had agreed to run a corrective ad, stating clearly in the headline that the ad was misleading.

But Dr. Simmons, suffused with some strange and inelegant sort of beneficence, took it upon himself to suggest that such gross and ungentlemanly phrasing might be out of order in dealing with the halls of Smith Kline & French and suggested the euphemistic headline: PUBLISHED AT THE REQUEST OF THE FOOD AND DRUG ADMINISTRATION TO REPLACE A PREVIOUS DYRENIUM ADVERTISEMENT IN THIS JOURNAL.

Not a word about "misleading," which Smith Kline & French had already accepted from Commissioner Edwards as a necessary slap on the wrist for their indulgences. No indication that the medical experts working under Simmons considered this "one of the most important ad cases" the

FDA had run into. It seems expressly clear that either Simmons was trying to be the white-haired boy of the drug industry, *or* he was stupid. But his academic and professional record could not possibly indicate that he was stupid.

Pinned down on his benevolent action on the part of Smith Kline & French, Simmons became the target of several penetrating questions from Congressman Fountain regarding the ad:

"It is not your opinion that it was not misleading?" the Congressman asked Simmons.

"No, sir," Simmons replied. "I think to some people it was misleading."

"Was it misleading to you?"

"I do not think it was intentionally so on the part of the people who put it together," Simmons said.

"Whether intentional or not," Congressman Fountain asked, "was it misleading?"

"Yes."

Dr. Goldberg added a question: "Regardless of what any physician on the outside might think or what you might think, is it not a fact that the FDA under Dr. Edwards' signature found it to be misleading?"

"Yes," said Dr. Simmons.

The same echoes of this situation keep repeating themselves constantly—the watchdog failing to be a watchdog. In some cases, he sleeps comfortably beside the fire. In others, he gets up and licks a hand. And it often appears, as far as the highest HEW and FDA echelons are concerned, the bigger the stranger, the softer the bark.

8

Rapidly Growing,
Frequently Troublesome,
Occasionally Tragic . . .

THE WORD around Washington is that the giant Drug Efficacy Study, finally completed in July, 1971, will have the biggest impact on the consumer of anything the FDA has sponsored in its entire history. The first results of the study hit the pharmaceutical manufacturers where they live, and their cries and wails are still echoing in the courts, laboratories, and lecture platforms through industry spokesmen.

The study began in 1966, when it became fully obvious that the FDA alone couldn't possibly review some 3,000 drug preparations still on the market from the days before the 1962 drug amendments went into force. With the help of the National Academy of Sciences, through its National Research Council, thirty panels of key physicians and scientists began the job of deciding whether the drugs involved were "effective," "probably effective," "possibly effective," or "ineffective." Since the panels were dealing with some of the sacred cows of the most sacred blue-chip companies, the jousting tiltyards at Camelot were hardly bloodier than the drug scene.

How could the situation be anything else, when *less than 20 percent* of the drugs reviewed were rated "effective"? The implication drawn from the FDA blacklist that summarized the study was that a massive number of people had been pouring a massive amount of money down the drain on drugs that doctors had been persuaded into prescribing—when the effectiveness of the drugs was less than proved.

Among the manufacturers represented on the list of drugs cited because they lacked substantial evidence of effectiveness or because their risk was greater than any possible benefit were some of the leading socialites of the drug business. But more alarming than that was the extensive number of their products that had been named by the FDA to be removed from the market:

E. R. Squibb & Sons	25
Eli Lilly & Company	23
The Upjohn Company	22
Charles Pfizer & Co., Inc.	17
Lederle Laboratories	15

Not that these were unique. Bristol Laboratories, Warner-Chilcott, Abbott, Wyeth, Parke-Davis, Merck, Sharp & Dohme, Colgate Palmolive, CIBA, Hoffman-LaRoche, Johnson & Johnson, Smith Kline & French were all represented, along with many others. What is most distressing is that none of these distinguished members of the Pharmaceutical Manufacturers Association had seen fit over the years to examine their own products and withdraw them from the market *before* the National Academy of Sciences-FDA effort forced them to do so. Such inaction gives a hollow ring to the protests the association launched as the study progressed.

In a carefully planned, well-coordinated campaign, the AMA and the PMA spread the word that the panelists on the Drug Efficacy Study were little more than "academic experts" who worked in "ivory towers" and who knew little or nothing about the "realities" of medical practice. This understandably raised the ire of Dr. William L. Hewitt, professor of medicine at the University of California medical school. He was chairman of the Panel on Anti-Infective Drugs for the study. He said:

"I have the responsibility for teaching medical students and young house staff physicians who for the most part will leave the University Medical Center environment well-trained for private practice. The major portion of this teaching is performed at the bedside of sick patients. Lest there be any misunderstanding I would like to emphasize that I am not an ivory tower basic scientist."

He went on to say that he had had a practice of his own for twenty years, which took up about a third of his time. In addition, he noted that most of the patients he saw were on the request of his medical colleagues.

Comments by panel members of the giant drug study indicate how flimsy much of the evaluation of the drugs had been in the past. Referring to muscle relaxants and drugs for the relief or prevention of vertigo, one NAS panelist commented: "I suspect that both classes of drugs have been exceptionally profitable to the drug industry, and I know that they have been extensively used by physicians, but with very little in the way of controlled clinical experiments to indicate their efficacy for the purposes which they are used."

Another member commented: "A study such as that just completed does bring home the fact that many drugs are being widely used with no or very little scientific justification."

Scores of other comments by the physicians participating in the drug review show many alarming reactions to the practices of the pharmaceutical manufacturers. Complaints regarding the paucity of good evidence for many "standard" drugs that had been used for years included phrases such as "surprise and dismay," "disturbing," "shocked," "really dreadful situation," "disheartened." Summing up his overall reaction, one disillusioned panelist concluded: "My reaction is strong to the effect that the drug industry had better learn how to conduct its own business in a proper manner."

One of the most startling and little-noted facts to come out of the study concerned the *ten most commonly prescribed drugs* in the United States today. *Seven* of these are noted in the report to *"either lack evidence for efficacy or are second or third choices for their purpose.* Of the remaining three, it is impossible to avoid the conclusion that they are vastly over-used. Of the ten drugs, only two are ordered by generic name."

These facts are a monumental tribute to the astute prowess of the pharmaceutical advertising and promotion men, a shocking commentary on the lack of real knowledge and the depth of naïveté on the part of the physician, and a tragic reflection on the kind of medication the American public is being saddled with by the drug companies.

The most intense storm center of the Drug Efficacy Study controversy, however, turned out to be the blunt and uncompromising ban on the "fixed combination" drugs. These are drugs previously mentioned that are made up of a mixture of ingredients, some of which might be duplicative, some might counter the action of others, or some might have too small a dose of one ingredient to be effective. They obviously were the major problem children of the study. *Half of the drugs reviewed were fixed-dose combinations*—1,500 of them. Very few were rated "effective."

This type of medication has been used in analgesics for the relief of pain, in drugs for rheumatic diseases, in obesity drugs, and in antibiotics. The latter group includes drugs like the infamous Panalba. Other fixed-combination antibiotics were made up of penicillin-sulfonamides, penicillin-streptomycin, and other antimicrobial agents.

Five panels studied this controversial question, aware that many of the drug makers have put these often expensive packages together as a sales gimmick and have added to their luster by hawking them from the rooftops to doctors who unfortunately continue to display a considerable capacity for gullibility.

The conclusion of all five panels is that these combination drugs are "ineffective as fixed dose combinations." Their conclusion goes on to indicate that the individual ingredients may be useful for specific diseases, but that no greater effectiveness can be expected from combining the drugs. Unanimously, the five panels agree that this type of therapy be discontinued.

Such drugs as penicillin and sulfa are at times dangerous

drugs, with severe and even fatal reactions sometimes reported. Using both drugs together compounds the felony and makes it almost impossible to tell which of the two drugs might be the villain in the case. Further, the doctor has no flexibility in increasing or decreasing the dosage of either ingredient, since the drug is locked into a fixed-combination format. One panel stated its case against Panalba in terms like this: "A large number of papers purporting to demonstrate clinical efficiency of this combination were reviewed. No properly controlled studies were located, and most consisted of reports of a few patients treated with variable results."

The panel on analgesic combinations was not much kinder. "There is increasing evidence," its report reads, "which has accumulated particularly within the past few years, that it is not always easy to predict the effects of adding one drug to another . . . [T]o promote such a mixture as an all-purpose remedy for all kinds of pain, including those which cannot possibly be aided by one or more of the ingredients, is, in the view of the Panel, to encourage bad therapeutics."

The panel on drugs used in rheumatic diseases was equally unfriendly: "The Panel feels strongly that the convenience to the patient in the use of a combination is heavily outweighed by the cited disadvantages, and it would favor disapproval of all the combinations that the Panel has reviewed."

As a result of the NAS action, an estimated $200,000,000 in questionable retail sales will go down the drain for the drug companies; conversely, the patient, as an unwilling guinea pig, will save a lot of out-of-pocket expense on ineffective and sometimes dangerous medicine.

With the lucrative market at stake on the combination drugs alone—to say nothing of the wider market that will be affected by the overall study—it is little wonder that the pharmaceutical companies are taking court action. So far, however, they have been unsuccessful. The FDA won its case against Panalba hands down, with the court holding that the FDA could ban a drug from the market without holding a special hearing. This is good news for the consumer but bad news for the drug companies, who in spite of their protests constantly assume the position of antagonist against him.

The repercussions of the study continue. Critical in the situation was the move by the Surgeon General of the United States, Dr. Jesse L. Steinfeld. He slapped a ban on all those products that were listed as "ineffective" and "possibly effective," * so that the use of these drugs by Medicare, Medicaid, and government hospitals and institutions would be a thing of the past.

The Task Force on Prescription Drugs of the Department of Health, Education, and Welfare summed up the entire problem of the Rx drug scene by saying that the citizens of this country deserve "the highest possible quality of health care, at the lowest possible cost." This is a situation much to be desired, but it is far from simple to achieve in the light of the roadblocks the drug makers throw in the way. Chief sufferers from their chauvinistic attitude are those over sixty-five.

The elderly are facing overwhelming medical and economic problems, with illness striking a large proportion of them and often throwing them into poverty because of it. What they have to pay for drugs takes large chunks of their incomes, which average only $70 a week. The amount they pay for prescription drugs is three times greater than for those under sixty-five. Out-of-hospital drugs are not covered by Medicare. Since only two of the ten most prescribed drugs are available under a generic instead of a brand name, most of the elderly have to pay an average of $4.11 for brand-name prescriptions instead of the $2.02 average for identical generic drugs.

Meanwhile, the brand-name drug manufacturers continue to cry poor, basing their arguments on the sums they pay for research and development. What they fail to mention is how much time and money they spend on molecular modifications on old drugs, which for the most part are the "me-too"

---

* Originally these were called "probably ineffective," but pressure on the FDA caused the wording to be changed.

drugs that do little or nothing more than create a useless patent so that they can charge more money for them. At the same time, the controversial fixed-combination drugs have been making up the vast majority of the so-called new drugs on the market. Even before the drug study, many hospitals, along with experts of the Armed Forces and on the drug study panels, found these inflated-price drugs to be unnecessary and duplicative.

An HEW task force found this burden placed on the ultimate consumer to be anything but an inexpensive fringe benefit:

> The task force finds that to the extent the industry directs a share of its research program to duplicative, noncontributory products, there is a waste of skilled research manpower and research facilities, a waste of clinical facilities needed to test the products, a further confusing proliferation of drug products which are promoted to physicians, and a further burden on the patient or taxpayer who, in the long run, must pay the costs.

Commenting on the inordinate amount that the prescription drug manufacturers spend on advertising and promotion—15 to 35 percent of sales—the same report said:

> Critics have asserted that intensive promotional efforts may be acceptable to sell such products as detergents, beer, and used automobiles, but not for such vital necessities as prescription drugs, that the expenses of drug marketing are excessive and add needlessly to the cost of prescriptions; that prescription drug advertising and other promotion has reached the proportions of supersaturation; and that some has been—at least until recent regulations were established by the Food and Drug Administration—inaccurate, unscientific, and biased.

The task force struck again at the detail men of the drug companies—20,000 strong—whose information for the doctor regularly includes lobbying propaganda and blatant oversell. As one former Parke, Davis detail man, now a pharmacist in a Connecticut town, said quite bluntly: "When I

went to call on a doctor, I told him about things I knew
nothing about—except by rote. Since he knew nothing about
what I was talking about, we were on very equal terms. That
made us comfortable. Just how comfortable the patient was
as a result of these talks, no one will ever know."

That the detail man was strapped into harness to lobby
against the Drug Efficacy Study is well documented. FDA
Commissioner Edwards had some telling words to say about
this after a large number of letters from doctors indicating
that the detail men were giving them considerable misinformation concerning the drug review. "Some of the information that has been disseminated to the physicians who have
written us has been supplied by drug detail men," he said.
"If this is the quality of what they are telling physicians
about the drugs they promote, we have a more serious problem with detail men than we thought."

There is an urgent need for direct communication between
government health authorities and the medical profession.
There is an urgent necessity for a better reporting system regarding adverse reactions to drugs. The number of people
who die from adverse reactions is simply not known. With an
estimated two billion prescriptions a year being written for
our overdrugged society, there is still no well-coordinated reporting system adequate to handle the situation.

About 20,000 adverse reaction reports a year from doctors
filter into the FDA, but experts figure this is a fraction of the
actual number, perhaps only 1 to 10 percent of them. The
new-drug explosion over the last three decades has created
almost an epidemic of adverse reactions, but no coordinated
"early warning system" has been set up, either nationally or
internationally. Without such a system, the stage setting for
another thalidomide disaster can always be possible, if not
likely. Much detective work on adverse reactions has been
done in retrospect, long after the fact, with many people
dying needlessly because no current system was available. It
took a study of those who had already died from venous
thrombosis and pulmonary embolism to pin down the dangers of oral contraceptives. No one yet knows what the long-

term use of the pills will bring. When hundreds of people were discovered to have died from asthma after using pressurized sympathomimetic aerosols, it wasn't until statistics assembled *after the fact* pinned down the cause. Many suspect that those who take analgesics such as aspirin or phenacetin regularly come down more frequently with urinary tract infections, but no widespread studies are available to confirm this.

If there had been a well-organized reporting system in effect, there might not have been the number of deaths that resulted from the irrational prescribing of "rainbow" diet pills—the regimen of combination of thyroid, amphetamine, diuretic, and digitalis pills sometimes prescribed for reducing. This form of treatment became popular when it was alleged that a patient could eat whatever he wanted and still lose weight. But because some drugs hid the harmful effects of other drugs in the "rainbow pill" program, the patient often failed to experience the symptoms that warn of damage being done to the body until it was too late. The FDA was able to force one of the major manufacturers of rainbow pills to stop selling thyroid and digitalis for the treatment of obesity, but not until considerable damage was done. In a warning about this type of program, the FDA said: "Overweight people should avoid so-called effortless weight-reducing schemes. Those who rely solely on drugs discover that they quickly gain weight again after they stop taking the medications. An individual who wants to lose excess pounds —and keep his health—must learn to limit the kind and amount of food he eats."

With so much confusion and acrimony among the professionals on the prescription drug scene, it is little wonder that the average consumer is more than confused. He needs the drugs that modern science has given him but is caught in the cross wind of the manufacturers' overwhelming lust for profit. He would like to know what new hopes are on the horizon, especially any major breakthroughs that might be coming up.

Not too much seems to be in the offing, or at least publicly announced. In 1970, L-dopa, the new drug treatment for Parkinson's disease, was pushed through on a crash FDA approval program, since nothing markedly effective had been available. This disease leaves its victims shaking with palsy, and up to 40,000 persons are hit each year, most of them over fifty. Because the benefits of L-dopa outweigh the risks involved, the FDA was able to process the applications of Hoffman-LaRoche and Norwich Pharmacal within three months. Heartening is the fact that some 65 percent of patients improved in overall clinical tests, although side effects can be severe.

Caution in enthusiasm for new drugs of great promise is always advisable. In early 1962 there was considerable fuss made over a drug labeled DMSO, which drew widespread interest because of its alleged pain-killing capacities and its uncanny ability to be absorbed through the skin. But by 1970 the drug still had not been approved for human use because of severe adverse reactions, especially involving eye changes in test animals. However, the drug is still under study for possible effectiveness in a variety of human diseases. In 1970 the FDA did approve its very limited use as an external treatment for horses to reduce swelling due to injury. A warning was included in the FDA statement that DMSO was not to be used on breeding stock or horses that were to be slaughtered for animal food purposes.

Any drug that purports to be effective against cancer naturally receives inordinate attention. Laetrile is one of these, and its merits have been argued in the press and elsewhere at considerable length. Laetrile is the brain child of an eighty-seven-year-old physician, Ernst T. Krebs, Sr., and his son, Ernst, Jr. They have never submitted a properly completed new drug application to the FDA. In 1962 they submitted two incomplete ones, and again in 1967 they requested investigational exemption for a new drug. About a year later the FDA had to turn this request down, because no preclinical studies had been completed with animal tests, as required. When the Krebses persistently shipped Laetrile for several years, the father and son were eventually clamped down on by the courts in both the United States and Canada.

No evidence has shown up that the drug is at all effective. The National Cancer Institute tested it against animal tumors, and the results were completely negative. Since the drug is derived from apricot kernels from California, that state's Cancer Commission investigated the drug and found it was totally ineffective in cancer treatment.

But the FDA is still willing to be convinced if the sponsors will back up their claims with well-controlled, scientifically conducted preclinical studies. Meantime, the FDA warns: "Laetrile should not be administered to humans under any circumstances."

Of less immediate impact but of greater long-term importance is the effect that drugs might have on generations to come. It is generally conceded by scientists that mutation, a basic change in the genes or chromosomes, is a major threat to human welfare. Nearly all mutations are harmful—up to 99.9 percent according to some estimates. They increase disease, create monstrous abnormalities, spread weaknesses, and increase malfunctionings. They can range from trivial, mild effects to death. Most mutations are mild—but they stay alive down through generations and spread to wider and wider sections of the population.

Most geneticists agree that we are accumulating mutations faster than they are being eliminated. As a result, the social burden is increasing. If the new and unknown by-products of drugs, food additives, and environmental hazards contain as many mutants as suspected, the accelerated mutation rate becomes an alarming threat. Neither the drug nor the food industry has shown evidence of respect for this problem to any extent.

Although the nature of mutation was clarified in the early 1920's, it wasn't until 1927 when it was discovered that X rays could create both gene mutations and chromosome breaks. It became obvious that X-ray radiation was something that had to be dealt with at arms length. In 1945 it was discovered that nitrogen mustard and mustard gas could bring about mutations in fruit flies. Other chemicals began to be suspect. But it wasn't until the major breakthrough of the discovery of deoxyribonucleic acid (DNA) that mutation could be studied right down to the basic molecule structure.

The discovery of the double helix model of DNA has brought science to the threshold of the possibility of creating and manipulating life. Some scientists feel that its discovery will have the greatest impact on man in all of history, far greater, for instance, than the splitting of the atom. And like the latter, it brings both fear and hope. Because DNA is the template that stamps out the program for every cell, every characteristic of the body, its manipulation can affect both the present and future generations—for good or bad.

John W. Drake, a geneticist speaking at the Conference on Evaluating Mutagenicity of Drugs and Other Chemical Agents in Washington in November, 1970, said: "If a certain amount of conservative genetic engineering can be coupled with wise environmental controls, it is within the foreseeable capacity of man to manipulate his own mutation rate to his advantage."

But this may be a long way off and extremely dangerous in the wrong hands.

One interesting fact emerging is that a large number of chemicals that cause cancer can also cause mutations, and the same is true in reverse. Concerned scientists are urging that drugs and food additives be routinely tested for their mutation-producing qualities in mammals before being approved by the FDA.

The importance of practical tests cannot be underestimated. W. L. Russell, at the Washington conference, urged an intelligent selection of these in order to "simplify the problem of estimating the hazards of a seemingly overwhelming array of potentially mutagenic chemicals in our environment."

The state of the union as far as drugs are concerned is anything but healthy. FDA figures show that up until the time that the new Drug Efficacy Study applied the brakes, at least, Americans were throwing away more than $500,000,-000 a year on prescriptions that showed no proof at all of being effective. Medical drug use is growing fast, but with little rationality. It is expected that sales of prescription drugs will soar some 50 percent over the next five years, to a staggering volume of three billion prescriptions annually.

Meanwhile, about 10 percent of the patients who take medication come down with adverse reactions, and half of them end up in the hospital either seriously ill or with their lives in danger. In the hospitals, 10 to 20 percent of the patients face the possibility of receiving the wrong medication. Physicians are prescribing far too many drugs to hospital patients, roughly eight to ten kinds per patient and sometimes up to thirty different varieties. The drug manufacturers continue to fight for the irrational use of fixed-combination drugs. Doctors in one part of the country treat the same disease with radically different drugs than in another, with little reason for the variation. In hospitals, further FDA figures show that over half of those patients treated with antibiotics showed no evidence of having a disease that needed that kind of treatment.

In a speech before the Academy of Pharmaceutical Sciences, FDA's Dr. Henry Simmons summed the situation up this way:

> We have a rapidly growing, frequently troublesome, occasionally tragic, and to a large extent needless and avoidable problem on our hands in the misuse of drugs in America. What can be more pathetic than to have an ineffective drug administered by error in a self-limited disease, with a severe or fatal drug reaction? I am not exaggerating the problem. We are at the point where we must realize that drugs are a mixed blessing, having much potential for good, but also some for harm.

9

The "Gras" Is Not Always Greener

IN THE early fall of 1969, the country was riding high on the Pepsi generation tide, to say nothing of diet Coke, orange, lemon and lime cyclamate-sweetened drinks that were being swilled down thirsty throats to the tune of about $1 billion worth a year. It was some six months before this that FDA's Dr. Jacqueline Verrett was looking at the thousands of pathetic chick embryos that had turned into grotesque little monsters from cyclamate injections. About 13,000 such embryos had been cataloged. Some had been injected with cyclamates. Of these, 15 percent showed the now familiar deformities of twisted or stunted skeletons, legs, and wings. Others had been injected with a cyclamate derivative. Of these, the score of malformations was 100 percent. Dr. Verrett's memo to the FDA Commissioner, Dr. Herbert L. Ley, Jr., made it very clear that there was a direct cause-and-effect relationship that couldn't be overlooked. But somehow that memo got lost. It never reached the Commissioner.

The full story of the cyclamate fiasco is actually as important today as it was then, because it precipitated the intensive review of all those substances that are being shoveled into the country's food supply by the profit-minded food industry and which are supposed to make up the "generally recognized as safe" (GRAS) list, mentioned earlier. GRAS additives, as they are called, are those that had been around before the food additive amendments of 1958. They include those chemicals which are considered by scientists and food experts as safe even when used over a long period of years or were generally accepted in food processing.

There are some 600 items on the GRAS list. Some of them are relatively innocent, like vinegar, pepper, and salt. They don't have to be cleared by the FDA before they are used as food additives. And, if you can believe the statements of such august groups as the National Canners Association, the Grocery Manufacturers of America, Procter & Gamble, and a considerable number of other leading food processors, the food manufacturers can make their *own* decisions as to whether a substance is GRAS or not.

Prominent on this GRAS list in the fall of 1969 were the cyclamates. As such, they could be dumped freely into Tab, Diet Pepsi, Fresca, Wink, Kool-Aid (nearly 30 percent cyclamate), Pillsbury Lime, Diet Delight Peaches, Metracal, candies, jams, jellies, ice creams, ice tea mixes, and kids' vitamin tablets. They enjoyed the same privileges as saccharin has held over the years. What makes the cyclamate story so applicable now is that the same story might be coming up as far as saccharin is concerned. Many other ingredients on the GRAS list that might carry unnoticed threats to the consumer are also suspect. The cyclamates had been kept on the market over the years, overlooked by all but a few. The potential for another cyclamate story is very real and possible, especially with saccharin, which is now assuming the cyclamate role.

Nobody took much notice when the use of cyclamates began to rise in the early 1960's. Consumption soared from 5,000,000 to 15,000,000 pounds over a four-year period. As the population counted calories, the beverage manufacturers counted profits, springing from the simple fact that it cost them some 60 cents for cyclamates against $6 for sugar for the same amount of sweetening power. Massive advertising and promotion campaigns for the diet drinks and foods pushed the tide along, so that near the end of the sixties, three households out of every four were filling up on products containing cyclamates. Everybody seemed to be forgetting that the original use of the chemical was supposed to be for very special diet needs of diabetics or pathologically fat persons. (Actually, there was great doubt that the chemical was either safe or effective for them.) Since cyclamates were on the GRAS list, no one had to clear them for safety with the FDA.

However, even in the middle fifties there was some slight concern expressed by the National Research Council of the National Academy of Sciences. The committee involved didn't seem to see any real danger in the chemical. But it did not feel there was sufficient data to show that children, pregnant women, or people with certain intestinal problems were altogether safe from adverse effects. By 1962, just when the mass use of cyclamates was taking off on an incredibly steep climb, the same NAS committee felt it had enough evidence to recommend that cyclamates be held down to exclusive use in special dietary foods. The committee's report stated flatly: "The priority of public welfare over all other considerations precluded, therefore, the uncontrolled distribution of foodstuffs containing cyclamates."

Neither the beverage and food manufacturers nor the FDA seemed to pay this any mind, except for some of the scientific personnel within the FDA whose voices went unheeded. What's more, by 1964 independent experts were voicing doubts not only about the safety of cyclamates but their value in controlling weight. The highly regarded publication *The Medical Letter* of September, 1964, took a hard slap at the vogue for diet drinks and foods engendered by rosy TV commercials that were as sickeningly sweet as the products they were pushing. The *Letter*, edited for physicians, added: "Even for weight reduction, the use of noncaloric sweeteners is of questionable value." Quoting a scientific study on the subject that found no significant difference between dieters on or off either cyclamates or saccharin, the *Letter* continued: ". . . the unrestricted use of artificial sweeteners makes little sense, especially since their safety is not beyond question. It should also be remembered that sugar is an important source of energy in children."

Most important in the *Letter* was its conclusion, especially since it was issued at such a critical time: "Until the many unanswered questions with respect to the toxicity of saccharin and cyclamate have been answered, *The Medical Letter* regards the current promotion and extension of use of these agents as against the public interest and believes that action by the medical profession, health authorities and Federal agencies to inform and protect consumers is in order."

This was in 1964, just as the diet drink companies flooded the market with their bottled cyclamates.

For a substance to be yanked off the GRAS list, it does not necessarily need to be proved harmful. The courts have indicated that if there is merely divided opinion among qualified experts, an ingredient cannot continue to be "generally regarded as safe." The manufacturer must then present convincing evidence that the product is safe. If there was any doubt that cyclamates were unchallenged by experts in 1964, it took little time for responsible scientific protests to grow.

A University of Wisconsin study in 1966 made it clear that there was a *sharp* difference of opinion about the safety of cyclamates and set the legal department of the FDA into action to figure out how to stall for more time in assessing the situation. By now the cyclamate sales thermometer had about doubled over the past four years and stood in the neighborhood of 12,000,000 pounds a year. Abbott Laboratories, as the largest manufacturer of cyclamates, was quite contented with the sales picture—but very wary of the rumblings against their pet chemical.

These were becoming louder, much louder. The same Wisconsin research group informed the FDA in the fall of 1967 that they were convinced from their studies that cyclamates should be ruled completely out of the food supply. In an internal FDA memo, one toxicologist wrote to a fellow associate: "We cannot say today that the cyclamates are generally recognized as safe; however, removing them from the GRAS list and establishing tolerances in soft drinks, etc., will produce difficult problems." But while the FDA was worrying about its "difficult problems," the consuming public was drowning itself in a sea of cyclamates, now moved up to the 15,000,000-pounds-a-year mark and still rising.

Hardly more than a month after this intramural memo was circulated, the Wisconsin group got together for a meeting with the FDA Commissioner. The minutes for the meeting were interesting in the light of the high administration stalling that was to happen later—and in view of the simple expedient that any difference of opinion among qualified experts should by law call for an automatic removal of a product from the GRAS list.

Referring to what the Wisconsin experts said at the meeting, the FDA minutes read:

> They felt they had now in their own laboratories and had seen sufficient other scientific results to lead them to the point where they should speak out in the public interest. They felt the cyclamates should clearly be removed from the GRAS list.
>
> Their first proposal was to limit the product to use in truly special dietary areas where nutritive sweeteners are contraindicated, but after further discussion of the possible harmful effects they believe have been shown, they changed their position to the point where the cyclamates should be ruled out of our food supply completely.
>
> They referred repeatedly to a cyclohexylamine [a derivative formed in the body from cyclamates] excretion and its passing of the placental barrier. They expressed a view that when pregnant women ingest cyclamates, their offspring may be born normal, but by the time of weaning they are somewhat stunted in growth and never catch up. They also expressed the view that there is mental disturbance in the child, as evidenced by some of their maze studies with animals.

In 1967 "difference of opinion" was obviously there—and many other places as well. But no action was taken by the FDA.

Nor was any action taken over a year later, on December 4, 1968, when another internal memo from a toxicological adviser in the FDA stated flatly: "The cyclamates should be removed from the GRAS status."

On the next day, the assistant director for Biological Sciences wrote: "It is obvious that our prior position regarding the safety of non-nutritive sweeteners should be altered. Current recognition of the relevance of subliminal pharmacology as a factor in chronic micro-insult by environmental factors dictates more than a passive attitude concerning these dietary adjuncts, especially the cyclamates which are now under closer scrutiny than the saccharins."

Two days after this was written, one National Academy of Sciences doctor wrote to another on his review panel: "As a minimum, cyclamates should be taken off the GRAS list. . . ."

Still no action. But the heavy promotional artillery barrage of the diet drink makers was continuing, and nearly three-quarters of the men, women, and children of the country were continuing to fill their stomachs with cyclamates, under the illusion that they were protected fully by the FDA from any lurking danger. Consumption of the chemical was approaching its high-water mark of 17,000,000 pounds a year.

On December 12, 1968, it looked as if the battle was over. A high-level FDA meeting on cyclamates reached several conclusions. One was that the FDA would undertake a public education program to warn against the unrestricted use of cyclamates. Another was that cyclamates would be removed from the GRAS list.

After this—silence. There was activity in the FDA, but little was heard about it. Dr. Marvin Legator was finding out that large doses of cyclamates clearly caused chromosome breakage in rats, with ensuing genetic damage. Dr. Verrett's chick embryo studies were continuing but hardly noticed. No public word was heard from the FDA about its clear-cut conclusion to remove the chemical from the GRAS list. Diet drink sales zoomed to nearly $1.5 billion.

Some eight months after the FDA meeting that reached the conclusion to ban cyclamates, in September, 1969, Paul Friedman, a TV journalist for the Washington NBC-TV outlet, decided to do some checking on the story. He had been prompted to do this when a friend of his refused a diet cola drink on the basis that he had heard some ugly rumors about the chemical and didn't want to take any chances. Friedman tracked down both Dr. Legator and Dr. Verrett and felt the information they gave him was worth a film segment on the local WRC-TV news show. He arranged for an on-camera interview with Jacqueline Verrett on the next day, September 30, 1969.

Dr. Verrett immediately checked with the FDA public relations office, and they and other officials arranged to be on hand for the filming of the interview. There was no suggestion to her that the interview was out of order, a point that was to come up with a vengeance when the storm broke later.

The interview was filmed September 30 for air use on October 1 on the local NBC station. Friedman had tried to interview Dr. Herbert Ley, FDA Commissioner at the time, but had been told on several occasions that he was not available.

Friedman shaped his story well. He indicated that many Americans try to fight weight in many ways, including the massive use of cyclamates. Then he introduced Dr. Verrett.

She showed some of the stunted chick embryos that had been treated with one of the cyclamates. The embryos were much smaller than the norm, with severe spinal deformities, and in some the foot was attached directly to the body at the hip. Others had a complete absence of the leg on one side. The echoes of the thalidomide tragedy were more evident than ever. But, as Dr. Verrett pointed out on the air, the cyclamates were not only causing the same abnormalities that thalidomide did in the chick embryos—they were causing more severe ones and in more frequent numbers. The interesting point here was that thalidomide had been used by only a few thousand pregnant mothers. Cyclamates were being poured into millions of homes in not only diet drinks but candy, canned fruits, medicines. "There is a higher incidence of malformation associated with cyclamate than with thalidomide under similar conditions of our experiments," Dr. Verrett told the television audience that night.

In order to balance his story, Friedman included a statement by Charles Brown, a scientist from Abbott Laboratories, the largest manufacturer of cyclamates. "The product has been around for twenty-five years, and other than a mild stool softening in human beings and some abnormalities in some species of animals not correlatable to man, we found no adverse effects of cyclamate as normally consumed by human beings," the Abbott spokesman said. Then he continued: "We would have no hesitation in saying that we would rate cyclamate and cyclamate-sweetened products as safe. . . ."

The Abbott spokesman did not mention the continuously growing doubts about the chemical on the part of leading scientists. Nor did he mention that the FDA several months before had agreed that cyclamates should be removed from the GRAS list. Why had they not been taken off when there were so many grounds over a stretch of several years? What was holding back the ban on cyclamates?

Paul Friedman ended his broadcast by saying that the chromosome damage and chick embryo tests raised disturbing questions about the safety of cyclamates, questions that had to be answered.

"But in the meantime," Friedman concluded, "cyclamates remain on the FDA's list of food additives generally recognized as safe. That means the government's position more closely reflects the views of business interests than it does the serious questions raised by FDA's own scientists."

The reaction was immediate. Commissioner Ley, responding to the broadcast, announced that he would ask the National Academy of Sciences to review the cyclamates—an obviously belated action. The Huntley-Brinkley network show carried by all NBC stations asked for a condensed version of Friedman's broadcast for the following evening. Notable was that Commissioner Ley claimed that he knew nothing about the results until learning of the TV interview.

The network broadcast was a mild, tamed version, keyed

to Ley's response rather than Dr. Verrett's tests. But it accelerated the momentum of the story.

The news broke across the board in the press, but most of the emphasis was still on Commissioner Ley's announcement rather than the ominous results of the research of both Dr. Legator and Dr. Verrett. Morton Mintz, of the Washington *Post*, noted caustically that Donald M. Kendall, president of Pepsi-Cola, the next day landed on the doorstep of Robert H. Finch, Secretary of Health, Education, and Welfare, under whom the FDA, of course, operated. Kendall, a close friend of President Nixon's and one of the leading buyers of cyclamates for his diet drinks, denied that the topic came up. Finch, however, had a different recollection. He said that he had brought the subject up in addition to other matters. Whatever the case was, Finch blasted his own FDA's scientist, Dr. Verrett, for speaking out of turn. He suggested that she had not cleared her interview with the proper authorities. Although it is uncontestable that she did clear with the correct channels, she had no chance to respond publicly to Finch's accusation.

On October 8, one week after reporter Friedman's newsbreak, officials from Abbott Laboratories tried once more to discredit all the adverse material that was accruing against its favorite chemical money-maker. But on this same day, Abbott also received news from an independent research laboratory that cyclamates had created cancerous tumors in rats it had under study.

Quite dramatically, the entire picture changed. Under the Delaney amendment, there is no option. The FDA must by law outlaw any substance in food that can create cancer in animal tests. The amendment does not apply to the terrifying results that Legator and Verrett had uncovered, since they were concerned with genetic problems rather than cancer. Congress had admittedly left this loophole some ten years before when it permitted administrative judgment to take the place of laboratory tests as far as any additive except the cancer-producing ones were concerned. But thanks to the Delaney amendment—which the food manufacturers are still trying to shoot down—the FDA was now forced to take action against the cyclamates, to take them out of food altogether rather than merely dropping them from the GRAS list.

By October 15, the National Cancer Institute had reviewed the results of the newly presented rat tests. There was no question about the results: The cyclamate-saccharin mixture used on the laboratory rats clearly induced cancer of the bladder. One unanswered question was why the Wisconsin cyclamate tests of the previous summer on mice, which produced the same bladder cancer, were not acted on promptly by Abbott. Although Abbott scientists knew about these tests, they chose to defend the indiscriminate use of cyclamates in food and drinks until they were forced into a corner with nowhere to turn.

The National Academy of Sciences review board, already in the middle of their own cyclamate review, was whipped into executive session on October 16 and 17, and the vote was unanimous that it was obvious that cyclamates could produce cancer in animals. All should have been over but the shouting.

But it wasn't. There now began another strange series of the Finch-industry incidents which even the most ardent defender of Finch's actions finds hard to defend. It began on the day of the major announcement, October 18, 1969.

Finch lost no time in taking a swipe at Dr. Verrett's work with the chick embryos, without mentioning her name. "I was unhappy," he said, "and expressed my unhappiness about the doctors in the Food and Drug Administration who chose in the case of the eggs, to go directly to the media without having even consulted with their superior, and with the office. That is not a procedure I approve, and it's certainly not acting in a very ethical way." He was joined in his condemnation of the scientist by Dr. Jesse L. Steinfeld, then Deputy Assistant Secretary of HEW, later Surgeon General.

But Dr. Verrett had gone to her superiors, including the FDA press office. Clearance had been obtained up through the Commissioner's office.

Then Finch did a very strange thing. Since the Delaney amendment blocked any action to keep cyclamate food products on the market, there was only one way this could be done: call them drugs instead of foods. The Delaney amendment did not apply to drugs, and the dodge was easy. Finch did just this in his announcement of October 18, a magic, overnight transformation. He ordered that "the artificial sweetener, cyclamate, be removed from the list of substances generally recognized as safe for use in foods." He went on to say: "I should emphasize also that my order does not require the total disappearance from the market place of soft drinks, foods, and nonprescription drugs containing cyclamates. These products will continue to be available to persons whose health depends upon them, such as those under medical care for such conditions as diabetes or obesity. I expect that in the future these products will be labelled as drugs, to be consumed on the advice of a physician."

After announcing his own thought about classifying cyclamate foods as drugs—an extremely strange procedure, to say the least—he set up a medical advisory panel to see how this odd rechristening could take place. The panel, meeting in November, barely a month after the explosive public announcement, came up with a report that said: "The use of cyclamates is not absolutely necessary in any disease, [but] it can be useful in the medical management of individuals with diabetes or patients in whom weight reduction and control is essential to health."

The medical group also added a few other things in its report. It noted that diarrhea could result from large amounts of cyclamates; that people's eyes were affected so that they were sensitive to light; that cyclamates affected and blocked many commonly used drugs; that they could cause excess loss of potassium from a patient using thiazide drugs; that the effectiveness of certain antibiotics could be reduced by the chemical. It noted also the cancer in rats and deformation of the chick embryos. Ironically, the cyclamates had been found to interfere with the action of diabetic drugs, used by the major group of people cyclamates were supposed to be helping. Further, pregnant diabetic women were particularly endangered by the cyclamates. One study showed that diabetic hamsters were especially susceptible to the cyclamate hazards.

But the medical report gave Finch what he wanted: an excuse to justify his initial statement about reclassifying the food additive into a drug. The pressures from the canning manufacturers to permit the use of cyclamates as far as canned goods were concerned was reported to be unbelievably strong. Close observers of the scene at the time say Finch went along with it, making an arbitrary decision in favor of the industry in opposition to the clear meaning of the Delaney amendment.

There was little question that the medical advisory group was hardly more than a smoke screen to justify a decision already made. The gut issue here was whether cyclamates could continue to be marketed under *any* conditions, even under the guise of "nonprescription drugs." This was a legal question, completely out of any medical group's competence.

The decision to permit this ploy created a comic opera situation. Food canners, such as Del Monte or Mott or Dole or dozens of others, now found themselves legally in the position of being drug manufacturers. Foods that had always been foods now found themselves being over-the-counter drugs. Finch's magic wand also would, if he was to get away with this maneuver, require that such canned foods or drinks be considered as *solely* for drug use. This, in turn, would shovel all of these products from the food bin and into the drug bin, where they would have to meet a whole different set of regulations.

To handle this chaotic situation, the FDA set about trying to legally justify Finch's decision—a decision which the FDA, not Finch, should have made in the first place. The first thing the FDA did was to make a simplified, special-privilege new drug application form for cyclamates. Immediately, strong voices of protest as to the legality of this rose up within the FDA. One internal legal document stated flatly: "To approve cyclamate-containing foods as safe and effective drugs within the concept of our enforcement of the new drug provisions of the Act is untenable. We are aware of *no* evidence that cyclamate-containing foods are safe or effective for use in the treatment of obesity or diabetes. Under the principles we strongly adhere to in permitting drugs to be marketed, these products should not be allowed on the market. To approve an NDA [new drug application] for these products is not supportable medically or legally."

The question at hand was: Were cyclamates both safe and effective—as all new drugs were legally required to be? Clearly, they were not, as Dr. John Jennings, FDA's Associate Commissioner for Medical Affairs, admitted when he said: "I would have to agree with the concept that we did not have substantial evidence that we usually require for the approval of a new drug."

In other words, what the FDA was doing was to try to support a political order from Finch, layman head of the HEW, and it was being hopelessly bogged down by the impossibility. There was no legal basis for cyclamates to continue to be foisted onto American consumers.

By the time that Congressman Fountain's subcommittee put the FDA administration on the carpet for all this chicanery, in June, 1970, Finch began beating a hasty retreat. He reconvened the same medical advisory committee, which now reversed itself. It cited as "additional" evidence an FDA report that showed that rats fed only one-sixth of the dosage used in the Abbott studies produced bladder tumors. This time, no saccharin was involved to cloud the issue. However, this study had been available to the medical group before it had whitewashed the Finch decision to permit cyclamates to stay around. Another study demonstrating damage to the cardiovascular system of laboratory animals was also available back in October. It was also cited at the time of reversing the decision as "additional" evidence.

The battle was over and Finch had lost—along with the billion-dollar industries that had been perfectly willing to keep on pouring a dangerous and treacherous chemical into its food and drink products, and the public be damned. A total ban was imposed on all cyclamates on August 27, 1970. Said Congressman Fountain after his probe into the matter: "Whether or not so intended, the action taken by the Food and Drug Administration clearly gives the appearance of being a subterfuge to keep cyclamates in foods and thereby circumvent the law."

But the cyclamate story, as a symbol of the entire consumer protection picture today, is not over. The food companies are still trying to weaken the Delaney amendment. Even though Nixon publicly called for the GRAS review on the heels of the cyclamate crisis, his administration continues to betray its gift of high priority for big business, low priority for the guinea pig consumer. The review of the 600-odd items on the GRAS list is becoming increasingly important, as the cyclamate story so graphically demonstrates. But big industry continues to fight it.

Senator Gaylord Nelson, pushing for the new Food Additive Safety Act, which will block use of additives without comprehensive pretesting, said: "Unless our food safety laws are vastly reformed, the American public will continue to serve as a massive testing ground for a variety of sweeteners, preservatives, spices, and coloring agents that are marketed without safety research. We simply must stop the practice of allowing food manufacturers to use the unknowing consumer as part of a large scale trial in the testing of food additives that have not been required to pass adequate laboratory examinations. Instead of weakening food additive laws (as the manufacturers are trying to do), we should broaden them to ban those additives that cause birth defects, mutations, and other biological damage as well as cancer."

With the end of the cyclamates, industry did the most logical thing—from its own point of view. It flooded the diet drinks, candies, foods, jams, ice creams with the old standby saccharin. Again, almost the same set of circumstances exists as it did with the cyclamates.

There is a strong difference of opinion among experts as to whether saccharin is capable of producing cancer or not. There are the same reservations about saccharin interacting with other drugs or chemicals to either block therapy or cause damage. A special panel of the National Academy of Sciences is studying the safety of saccharin for use in foods, just as it was doing with cyclamates. Its provisional report spoke not much better, if as well, as the previous NAS report on cyclamates. The report called for an examination of patterns of saccharin consumption, tests for the chemical's cancer-producing qualities, and a further look at how saccharin interacts with other drugs. "None of these recommended studies have been fully carried out," the report stated.

Under these conditions, it is logical to wonder why the diet drink and food companies have plunged so heavily into replacing cyclamates with another potentially dangerous product. Again, the situation is this: Any nonnutritive sweetener had as its original purpose the amelioration of the unfortunate few who suffer from diabetes* or pathological obesity, where the benefit might possibly outweigh the risk. Even this, however, is uncertain. With the mass-market sale and wild promotion of products like diet drinks, the picture changes measurably. Pregnant women, infants, children, teen-agers, the aged and infirm—all types of people use the product on a wide and uncontrolled scale. The dangers are radically increased further because there is no medical supervision. To rush from cyclamates into saccharin, where again three out of every four Americans are exposed to the chemical, can, according to some scientists, be equal to jumping from the frying pan into histology labs. But, for the comfort of the food and drink producers, saccharin is so much cheaper than sugar.

There is already a well-documented study showing that rats suffer malignant bladder tumors when a pellet mixed with cholesterol and saccharin has been implanted in their bladders, just as with cyclamates. There are already tests by Dr. Verrett with chick embryos showing the same results

* A radical change, however, has taken place. In a dramatic announcement in October, 1971, the American Diabetes Association recommended that doctors permit their diabetic patients to use sugar just as ordinary people do.

with saccharin as with cyclamates. Another study shows that saccharin increases the toxicity of insulin in rats—and insulin is the best friend of diabetics. These, in turn, would be the most likely to use saccharin frequently.

The NAS panel admits that two long-term saccharin feeding tests that failed to create cancer in rats and mice were inadequate in the light of recent developments in bladder and kidney pathology. In another test purporting to indicate that saccharin was reasonably safe, only five out of the forty rats present at the start lived through to the end of the test. Yet in spite of these and other thunder clouds on the saccharin horizon, the NAS panel concluded in 1970 that the present and projected use of saccharin did not pose a hazard. Again, it appeared suspiciously like the cyclamate story.

The specter of the NAS panels being frequently dominated by industry personnel and sympathizers still continues. It is impossible to tell how many members of the panels receive large consulting fees from industry or who own stock in the companies they are supposed to be regulating. For instance, in 1971 the chairman of an NAS committee on cereal products was from Continental Baking Company. The chairman on a committee on microbiology of foods was from the H. J. Heinz Company. The chairman of a committee on containers was from Reynolds Metals. The president of the NAS Agricultural Research Institute was from the National Canners Association, notorious for its resistance to consumer protection legislation.

The panel that reviewed the saccharin evidence in 1970 reflects a clear pro-industry viewpoint. There is no evidence that it is directly under the thumb of industry. Its views, however, are challenged vigorously by the Wisconsin scientist Dr. George T. Bryan, whose cyclamate tests revealing the bladder cancers were so critical in the ultimate ban of cyclamates. "It would appear most prudent at this time to limit saccharin utilization to diabetics, the severely obese and others with specific medical need," he told a *Wall Street Journal* reporter. "To do other than this might result in the needless exposure of many individuals to a potential carcinogen."

Dr. Bryan's conclusions were that the same problems with cyclamates were clearly evident with saccharin—and the Food and Drug Administration was derelict in its duty in not slapping a ban on saccharin as it had done with cyclamates. Speaking to reporters at an American Cancer Society's seminar, he said: "I don't know how the FDA was clairvoyant enough to ban only the cyclamates."

The FDA claimed at this point that it had been assured by the National Academy of Sciences that there wasn't any immediate danger from the amount of saccharin being consumed by the public. However, this is also almost exactly the same situation as with the cyclamates. Dr. Bryan's pellet implant tests revealed saccharin as being capable of producing cancer in animals. The only thing blocking a full ban on saccharin under the Delaney amendment was the technical argument about the word "ingested." Enough scientists claimed that planting pellets inside an animal was not "ingesting" the chemical—even though Dr. Bryan disagreed. But he also pointed out that the Abbott tests (that eventually caused the cyclamates to be banned) were based on a mixture of cyclamates and saccharin. Why, he asked, were not both chemicals banned? The question remains unanswered. And to punctuate his comments, Dr. Bryan felt that the negative evidence is strong enough to inspire him to remove all products containing saccharin from his household.

Another incident arose in July, 1971, that raised even more questions about saccharin, which has actually been under doubt and scrutiny since the days of Theodore Roosevelt. At that time, the food industry opposed any attempt to squelch the profitable item. In the recent incident, the National Academy of Sciences review panel suggested a 100-to-1 safety ratio for use of the product. Through what FDA's Virgil Wodicka called a mathematical error, this ratio has been dropped to 30 to 1—a considerably softer stand for the food manufacturers and one which, strangely enough, would not cause any reformulation of diet foods and beverages.

At this writing the saccharin question is wide open, again dramatizing the importance of the full-dress GRAS review, which, for good or for bad, will have a profound effect on the consumer for years to come.

10

The Mighty Micro-Insult

THE WORD "micro-insult" is an interesting one. When it comes to food additives, it's critical. It represents the massive number of small insults the human system is exposed to, not from any gigantic assault of grossly harmful artificial substances, but from the persistent, continuous, undramatic bombardment of the four pounds of artificial colors, chemical preservatives, so-called stabilizers, and flavorings each of us absorbs each year as a gratuity from the food manufacturers. This four-pound package is an imposing mass of varied materials. It consists of more than 3,000 chemicals that are tossed into the food we eat. Even if many of them are reasonably safe, there's not a scientist living who can say with certainty what happens when they combine with each other or pile up on top of each other.

In fighting the Delaney amendment, the manufacturers claim that "safe limits" could be set, even for those chemicals that are known to produce cancer. What they don't mention is that while one food might have such a small amount of a cancer-producing chemical in it that it might be harmless, a dozen or more other foods or drinks might have the same additive. The micro-insults might well add up to a major tragedy.

What's more, the same type of chemicals that are put into foods might also be absorbed unknowingly from the environment, or from direct medication, or from medicines that are fed to animals that are later eaten by man.

From the point of view of protecting or increasing the food supply, there is no question that many additives are important. The problem comes from the gross disregard of the collection of micro-insults that are increasing in this synthetic age. The cumulative effect can be harrowing unless restraints are imposed.

The review of the GRAS list by the National Academy of Sciences assumes a special importance at this time. Scores of these "generally regarded as safe" products have *never* been tested. They have been having a free ride on the basis that they have been around for a long time. Most additives are put into foods for one basic, driving reason: They bring more profits. If there is any doubt, the toss of the coin should favor the consumer rather than the manufacturer.

The GRAS list is a boon to the manufacturer because he doesn't need to go through the painfully slow process of filing a petition with the FDA to clear the substance before packing it into his product. What has happened, however, is that modern research methods are showing up hidden dangers that were impossible to detect before. In addition, new types of foods, like the textured protein products that simulate meat, are demanding increased use of the old standby GRAS products and other additives. Nobody knows what dangers lie in this.

The most optimistic forecasts for the completion of the GRAS review indicate 1974 or 1975. Meanwhile, the consumer will go on being a guinea pig as the manufacturers go on fighting to keep whatever profit-making chemicals they can in their products.

Within the last ten years, the use of food additives has gone up about 50 percent. In a single cake mixture you can find bleaches, antioxidants, emulsifiers, enzymes, color additives, artificial flavorings, preservatives, spices—to say nothing of the leftover mercury fungicide and parathion insecticide residues clinging to the flour, along with a fumigant to add to the feast. On one of the first *Great American Dream Machine* shows over the NET network, biting satire was broadcast with actor Marshall Efron as a modern-day chef. (NET, it seems, is the only network with courage enough to blast the food industry, or any industry. It has no sponsors, as other networks do.) In a laboratory setting, Efron stood behind a counter with all the chemicals that went into making up a Morton's Lemon Cream Pie. Then he proceeded to mix the chemical ingredients from assembled test tubes, stirring them into a formless glob of matter.

The micro-insults included sodium caseinate, monosodium glutamate and diglycerides, monosodium phosphates, modified food starch, gelatin, whey solids, dextrose, lecithin, sodium bicarbonate, guar gum, ammonium bicarbonate, and several other assorted chemicals.

At the completion of the segment, he held up a package of the Morton product and pointed out that here was a factory-fresh pie—no lemon, no cream, but all the same a Morton's Lemon Cream Pie. It was a bitter, ironic, and altogether true commentary on the present-day food scene. Not one peep of protest emerged from the pie manufacturer, because everything used in the sketch consisted of the actual chemicals, and nothing in the sketch was false.

Efron's similar treatment on what he called creative play-foods was no less irreverent. "Here's an old favorite of kids everywhere," he told the NET television audience. "Fumaric acid, sugar, propylene, artificial flavoring, calcium carbonate, and every school boy knows the rest. Kool-Aid—no muss, no fuss, and no fresh fruit leftovers to clean up and throw away. This little packet delivers two quarts of non-nourishing, imitation-flavored soft drink. All you do is rip open the packet, toss the contents into a non-metal pitcher, add more sugar, cold water, stir, and serve. A non-metal pitcher; I wonder what it would do to a metal pitcher?"

He went on to point out that Kool-Aid was one of the winners in the price battle—coming to over $5.00 a pound. But this was nothing, he later added, compared to McCormick brand chives, which would mount to $103.68 per pound.

That's where the expression "worth his weight in chives" comes from, he informed his viewers.

Ominous in implication and dramatizing the importance of the new GRAS review is the statement by Dr. Joshua Lederberg, a Nobel laureate in genetics. On the heels of the cyclamate crisis, he said: "There are surely dozens of compounds already approved for use which will prove to be at least as hazardous as cyclamate, but have yet to reach the same kind of attention."

The big question as far as the consumer is concerned is whether or not he will be getting his tax money's worth in the National Academy of Sciences GRAS review. Will the review panels be under the thumb of industry? Will they be like Secretary Finch—soft and easy on the assessment of possible dangers?

Industry has garnered a lot of arguments to try to hold back rational assessment of the additive hazards. The big trade associations are constantly pointing out that the high doses of a chemical given to laboratory animals has no meaning as far as man is concerned. Dr. Umberto Saffiotti, of the National Cancer Institute, struck out at this theory by saying: "If we have something that produces cancer in 10 percent of the animals tested at levels of consumption that are, say, 10 times higher than those we see in man, we could possibly infer that this might produce cancer in man, with the frequency of one-tenth of what we see in animals. We would have an incidence, possibly, comparable to 1 percent in man. It is a very high risk. Now, are we willing to settle for something like that? I say we shouldn't."

Another bromide the manufacturers like to noise about is that there is such a thing as a "safe" level for an additive, even if it does cause cancer in larger amounts.

Here, the micro-insult comes into play, where a cumulative collection of the substance goes to work with a vengeance. The sophistry of the manufacturer has a particularly hollow ring under these conditions. His efforts to get rid of the Delaney amendment can only result in increased danger to the consumer. Delaney had to fight to keep his amendment in the 1958 laws when they were evolved. The "zero tolerance" for any cancer-producing additive is one of the consumer's best protections today. The World Health Organization fully subscribes to this safeguard. Those who argue that there was no evidence that the cyclamates had caused cancer in man failed to consider that large-scale use of the chemical held sway for only about seven years. Experts consider that it takes almost twenty years for cancer to show up from a direct cause. What hangover will show up from the big diet drink jag two decades or so from now?

Perhaps one of the most frequent arguments bandied about by the food industry is that *any* chemical fed to animals in large enough doses would produce cancer. This is simply not true. In one study by Bionetics Research Laboratories, mice were fed with the highest possible doses they could take and still stay alive. Only 25 percent of over 100 chemicals tested produced any tumors. Many other tests indicate the same type of result.

The same argument is used by industry in its attack on animal tests that show that a substance causes mutations. Some critics have claimed that *any* substance could cause them. Yet Dr. Cecil Jacobson, of George Washington University, has shown that of 275 substances tested for mutation-producing possibilities, only 7 did so. In another test of 100 substances, only 6 produced positive results.

Most important in the new GRAS review is that most of the items will be examined not only for their cancer-producing potential but for their capacity to bring about birth defects and changes in the genes. In the chemical age we are living in these dangers are becoming increasingly serious. They are not covered by the Delaney amendment. Additives which are capable of producing birth and gene defects are now permitted if a "safe level" can be determined.

Again, the micro-insult comes into play. Any continuous piling up of these agents through their inclusion in many *different* foods and drinks can be dangerous. The fight looming in this area is between Congress and big industry. The latter wants to remove the Delaney amendment entirely. Senators

Nelson and Ribicoff are pushing for it to be extended to bar any additives that can cause birth defects, mutations, and other biological damage. The battle is a real one. Who is on the side of the angels and who represents the enemy of the people is obvious from the consumer's point of view. The pattern is consistent, whether it is drugs or foods.

The loophole in the law that permits the use of food additives that are capable of causing birth defects and gene damage seriously threatens the future of the country. Three expert committees have recommended legislation be passed to protect the consumer, but none has yet been passed.

The new GRAS review study got off to a shaky start in December, 1970. There was considerable dissension in both the FDA and its parent, the HEW, as to how the study was to be announced publicly. Several officials felt that it was a very hot issue and that great care had to be taken when it was presented to the press and broadcast media. The cyclamate story was still fresh in everyone's mind, and there were two specific items that nearly everyone was interested in: saccharin and monosodium glutamate. The rumbles about both of these common additives being taken off the "safe" list were loud and frequent. The FDA was not at all keen about answering embarrassing questions about them, since there was little conclusive they could say.

A tricky area that was bound to come up and bite the manufacturers were those items that the manufacturers had claimed to be generally recognized as safe but had no official FDA sanction. These are items which Jim Turner, author of *The Chemical Feast*, called the gray list. Turner pointed out in his book that FDA's Deputy Commissioner Winton B. Rankin said in 1969: "The manufacturer is entitled to reach his own conclusions, based on his scientific evidence that a subject is, in fact, generally recognized as safe. And he is not required to come to us, then, and get the material added to the list." This, said Turner, led only to disaster. "Since, in Rankin's words," Turner wrote, "the industry is not required even to tell the FDA which items it is assuming are safe, there is no possibility of systematically checking the safety of these items. For all practical purposes, the FDA has relinquished control of food additives to industry."

When Jim Turner led the research group from Ralph Nader's Center for the Study of Responsive Law into its investigation of the Food and Drug Administration, the FDA was totally unprepared for what would follow. The group consisted of a swarm of perceptive, dedicated university students, and they began with the bottom ranks of FDA activity and worked slowly up to the top. When they reached the top administrators, they were armed with such massive information that the Nader group tripped up the top brass consistently in their attempt to explain away the failures of the agency in protecting the consumer from the onslaughts of big industry. When Herbert Ley, then FDA Commissioner, testified before a Congressional committee on monosodium glutamate (otherwise known as MSG, and principally marketed as Accent), Nader and Turner's study group picked up five glaring errors in his testimony.

What the Nader study group did in uncovering the venality of the baby food manufacturers not only demonstrates the FDA's frequent attitude of permissiveness to industry (much of it traced to the White House love affair with big industry) but also dramatically documents the incapacity of industry to police itself—as if that needs any more evidence than is glaring out through the pages of food and drug history.

Both Gerber and Heinz came under the Nader study spotlight. The study uncovers a letter to Gerber stockholders regarding the George Washington University research that showed that MSG injected under the skin of two- to ten-day-old mice clearly caused brain damage. The research concluded that "so long as there is any doubt as to the safety at all, I think it the better part of prudence not to have MSG in baby food." Lamenting that Dr. Jean Mayer, nutrition adviser to the President, was denouncing the use of MSG in baby foods, the Gerber stockholder letter, in a series of half truths and distortions, tried to blame most of the consumer disquietude on Nader's TV appearances and other press coverage of the story.

Jim Turner blasted Gerber's basic contention that a food additive can remain on the market until it is definitely proven to be dangerous, pointing out that the intent of the law is that an industry must establish the safety of an additive *before* using it. "Clearly MSG should not be used in baby food and should have been removed as soon as doubts were raised about its safety," Turner said. "It was not removed until October, 1969, five months after the report of the brain damage, three months after Senate hearings on the potential danger, and one day after Dr. Mayer denounced the use of MSG in an address. It is not clear that MSG would have been removed from baby food without public pressure, which means that the FDA, which should have taken legal action to force the removal, was not doing its job."

One of the snider memos the Nader and Turner study unearthed was in the form of a telegram from the president of International Minerals and Chemical Corporation (makers of the Accent brand of MSG) to the chairman of the Food Safety Panel of the White House Conference on Food, Nutrition, and Health:

MR MURPHY OF CAMPBELL SOUP HAS TOLD ME OF YOUR INTEREST IN SEEING THAT THE UPCOMING WHITE HOUSE CONFERENCE ON NUTRITION IS KEPT WITHIN BOUNDS OF ITS STATED PURPOSE AND THAT IT NOT BE USED FOR RUBBER STAMPING THE UNREALISTIC THOUGHTS AND PROPOSALS OF COMPLETELY UNINFORMED AND BIASED SO-CALLED PROTECTORS OF THE CONSUMER. . . . AS THE NATION'S LEADING PRODUCER OF MSG WE KNOW FULL WELL THE MAGNITUDE OF THE TASK. WE HAVE FOR EIGHTEEN MONTHS FOUND OURSELVES IN THE POSITION ONE TIME AFTER ANOTHER OF BEING TRIED BY THE PRESS ON THE UNJUSTIFIED AND TOO OFTEN UTTERLY DISTORTED STATEMENTS OF NOT ONLY PSEUDOSCIENTISTS, BUT THOSE IN GOVERNMENT CIRCLES WHO SOUGHT POLITICAL FAVOR WITH THE PUBLIC THROUGH ASSOCIATION WITH THE SO-CALLED CONSUMER PROTECTIONISM.

WE HAVE IN EVERY INSTANCE HAD TO PROJECT OURSELVES AGGRESSIVELY INTO THE PICTURE TO PRESENT THE TRUE FACTS, FIRST TO BE HEARD BY THE SENATE SELECT COMMITTEE ON NUTRITION AND HUMAN NEEDS, WHEN MONOSODIUM GLUTAMATE

[MSG] BECAME A TARGET AS AN INGREDIENT OF BABY FOODS, A
NATIONAL EMOTIONAL MEDIUM FOR GARNERING PUBLICITY, AND
SECOND, WHEN THE FLURRY OF PUBLICITY ON CYCLAMATES
RESULTED IN MSG BEING DRAGGED ONCE AGAIN INTO THE CONSUMER
SPOTLIGHT ON THE BASIS OF LIMITED AND INCONCLUSIVE
EXPERIMENTS BEING TAKEN AS PROVEN FINDINGS AGAINST A
QUARTER OF A CENTURY OF TRUE SCIENTIFIC RESEARCH.

It is obvious that such a telegram not only borders on paranoia but that it demonstrates a gargantuan disregard for consumer interests. Twice it refers to "so-called" consumer protectionism, as if this were one of the cardinal sins of the nation. And if a "consumer protector" is biased on the part of the consumer, what better bias could he have? Which is more important? The consumer or International Minerals? Should a "consumer protector" favor profits over consumer health and safety? Other industry spokesmen have referred to the consumer who wants protection as being "sinister" and applying "terrorism" and "blackmail," as Jim Turner points out. Restraint for the safety of the consumer on the part of the manufacturer is such a simple premise. Why do the manufacturers fight it?

The Nader study uncovered the story of Dr. Thomas A. Anderson, former chief of the Heinz Nutritional Research Laboratory, who made the mistake of suggesting to his company that it change some of the materials in its baby foods because their quality was shoddy and their potential danger had not been assessed. Heinz refused, on the basis that it would hurt its competitive position, and then went about trying to stop Dr. Anderson from testifying before a Senate committee on nutrition.

Jim Turner went on to indicate several other weaknesses in FDA's control of the food-chemical revolution. Bacon preserved by atomic radiation for unrestricted public consumption, for instance, was approved by the FDA in 1963—then was withdrawn when rat and dog deaths shot up when the bacon was tested on them. Folic acid, a nutrient; NDGA, the antioxidant for fatty foods; oil of calamus, for flavoring candy, baked goods, beverages, etc.—all had been approved at one time by the FDA, then later withdrawn when it became apparent they could cause damage. NDGA, the brominated vegetable oil, had caused mesenteric cysts and kidney lesions in rats, as did other oils of the same type. These brominated oils were favorites of the citrus fruit drink makers and were not removed from the GRAS list until April, 1970, when they were quietly squelched. The only reason, say some authorities, that this withdrawal from the market failed to make as large a splash as the cyclamate ban was that the brominated oil market was only a fraction of the size of the cyclamates.

With the announcement of the GRAS review, Ralph Nader and his Center for the Study of Responsive Law hit strongly at the FDA's failure to require toxicity tests for all synthetic items on the GRAS list. He pointed out that there had never been any laboratory tests on many of the items on the list and that simply a review of the meager literature available would be meaningless. He also hit at the FDA's proposal for "interim" clearances for some substances, claiming that such a procedure was not within the law. Further, Nader emphasized that consumers were not represented in the GRAS review, while industry's Flavor and Extract Manufacturing Association had been invited to help evaluate the very products that provided extra profits for its members.

Of course, the FDA was also hit from the other side of the fence. Kraft, General Mills, Campbell Soups, Nestlé, and other food processors all protested about the various hardships they would have to undergo if the GRAS list were cut down. Other firms were concerned about giving away trade secrets to the FDA—an understandable complaint, except that when public safety is at stake, there can be little compromise if maximum protection is to be assured.

The GRAS review was faced with the same problem as its sister Drug Efficacy Study: The review consisted mainly of going over old-hat material that had been around for years and did not anticipate many fresh studies under active laboratory conditions and with the use of updated techniques.

What's more, practically all of the basic information the
FDA requires has to come from industry itself.

From the point of view of the consumer, FDA's Dr. Virgil
Wodicka's attitude toward what he called conscious food additives—additives intentionally put into foods by the makers
—is puzzling. By putting this problem last on his list of urgent priorities, he seemed to fail to regard the warnings of
credible scientists who were showing a lot more concern and
alarm about the cumulative effect of such rapidly multiplying food engineering.

Referring to the possibility that any previously innocent
additive might be ruled out suddenly and unexpectedly, he
said: "There always exists the possibility that one more test
will rule the material out, particularly under an arbitrary
legal criterion. [He was referring, of course, to the Delaney
Amendment, which barred *any* cancer-producing additive.]
There is nothing that can be done to guard against this con-
tingency."

There is an interesting attitude revealed here. By calling
the Delaney Amendment an "arbitrary legal criterion," he
suggests reluctance to go along with this important legislation, which he is hired to enforce.

Both Wodicka and men like Howard Bauman, a vice-president of Pillsbury, seem inclined to regard the protests
against the piling up of additives into foods as a scare campaign. "Industry must accept some of the blame," Bauman
told a Senate hearing, "because of its silence in the area of
food additives." Then he went on to say: "There's no question that the scare stories about food additives and accusation that the food industry is processing out all the good has
provided a fertile field for the proponents of the 'natural.'"

There is little wonder that the public was paying more attention to natural foods. If industry showed more evidence of
restraint or concern for the consumer's safety, the trend
might not be so strong. The case for additives can be rational
in many cases, provided that industry shows more of a pro-
clivity to check for safety before it uses them, rather than
after.

Critics of the new FDA GRAS review pointed out that its new definition of the word "safe" shifted the burden of proof away from the manufacturer, since an item could be considered GRAS as long as it didn't show any evidence of being a hazard. The ubiquitous Jim Turner faulted this definition, calling for industry to prove that an item is safe before use.

In contrast to this, the equally ubiquitous Abbott Laboratories, whose record on both the food and drug scenes might inspire a more discreet silence, spoke out loudly against the FDA review proposals. Abbott came out flatly against the whole idea and argued that the FDA proposal simply be abandoned. In a submission of its stand to the FDA, Abbott said the FDA proposal "should clearly indicate that the manufacturer has the right and duty to make a determination of whether a substance is in fact GRAS." Coming on the heels of its role in the cyclamate story and in the middle of its intravenous fluid problem, the statement seemed rather off key.

Industry reactions such as this were instrumental in drawing the attention of members of both House and Senate.

"The American people," Senator Ribicoff said, "have generally assumed that new food additives have been tested by the government and licensed as safe. This proves to be anything but the case. . . ."

Senator Humphrey, a member of the same Senate subcommittee, joined Senator Ribicoff to call for hearings on "chemicals and the future of man." Humphrey was also incensed by the industry spokesmen who had claimed the right to add chemicals and other substances to foods without letting either the FDA or the consumer know about it. This, he said, was a public-be-damned attitude. "The FDA has not been strong enough in policing the use of additives, and its reaction to these recent industry statements sounded like an apology for the food companies," he said.

Senator Ribicoff's Subcommittee on Executive Reorganization and Government Research lost little time in getting at the root of the problem. Within a few months after industry's uncompromising statements, hearings began to explore and analyze every possible phase of "chemicals and the future of man."

The questioning and the testimony bore down on three basic questions that were predominantly on the minds of most thinking consumers: How much do we really know about the hazards to human health from these food-engineering chemicals? How much assurance of safety do we need? What can the federal government do to make sure these chemicals we absorb are safe?

The subcommittee, utilizing months of painstaking research by Robert S. Bird of the professional staff, began working on the assumption that the cyclamates had been only the tip of the iceberg. There were a great many straws in the wind that suggested the validity of this assumption: the synthetic estrogens that remained in meat; various food dyes and coloring that were being put under careful scrutiny for their cancer-producing potential; and, of course, the suspicious preliminary findings on saccharin, to say nothing of nitrites, used so frequently in processed meats.

The committee probed not only the cancer dangers but the birth and gene defects that might arise from the cumulative effects of the sustained eating of the 800,000,000 pounds of the 3,000 different chemicals deliberately added to our foods.

And what about the $60 billion worth of convenience foods, including TV dinners, snack, and frozen foods? And, of course, the GRAS list. Why did the National Academy of Sciences state that an informal "GRAS appraisal can provide assurance of safety sufficient to obviate the need for subjecting every food chemical, irrespective of its origin, to the extensive animal testing required to support a food additive petition?" To the subcommittee, this kind of thinking seemed particularly specious in view of what had developed in the cyclamate situation.

Further, since most chemicals are added to benefit the profits of the seller, why shouldn't the proof of safety be required before marketing rather than after? Should the health risk to the consumer be put after the economic benefit of the seller? What about the gaping hole that remains in the law to permit the most harmful chemicals as far as genetic damage is concerned to slip untested into the market? Why doesn't food chemical testing require the kind of clinical research that drugs must undergo?

Key man in the investigation was Dr. Samuel S. Epstein, of the Children's Cancer Research Foundation and the Harvard Medical School, a highly regarded and outspoken scientific expert on the effects of food chemicals on the human system. His conviction was that the consumer protection laws should anticipate the dangers rather than discover them afterward, such as with the cyclamates.

He divided the synthetic chemicals that get into our food into two classes. The first is the intentional, the chemicals that are deliberately added to the food to improve quality, texture, and color—the latter two being mainly of cosmetic value. The second he regarded as accidental food additives, such as DDT and other pesticides and heavy metals like mercury.

In addition to the growing concern about cancer-producing chemicals and those that produce gene and birth defects, Dr. Epstein considered the very real possibility, as yet unexplored, of chemicals we are exposed to that may produce psychobehavioral effects. Added to that is another unexplored area—those chemicals that can break down the immunity of the body's defense mechanisms.

Dr. Epstein had little patience with those who argued that the economic benefits warrant risking the health of any consumer. One malformed child can cost the state around $250,000 for medical care alone. If future generations are affected by chemical-induced malformations over the years, the cost is simply uncountable.

There are other ironies of the frequently sounded benefit-to-risk theory industry likes to uphold. DDT is a cancer-producing pesticide. Its major use in this country is for control of insects that attack cotton. But these insects are generally resistant to the pesticides. Is there any benefit to match this risk? Or another pesticide, Mirex—it, too, produces cancer.

Yet it is being used for fire ant control. This insect shows no
evidence of creating a hazard for man or animal. What is the
ratio of benefit to risk? Ironic also is the fact that up until
mid-1972 we continued to use DDT when there were adequate substitutes that are nontoxic and nonpersistent.

Many conditions, including cancer, birth defects, and
changes in the genes, that once were considered spontaneous,
Dr. Epstein revealed, are actually brought on by food and
environmental hazards. Weak carcinogens are more trouble
for the scientists to detect than the obvious strong ones, like
aflatoxins and nitrosamines. There is evidence that air pollution gives cancer a considerable boost. If you live in a city
and you smoke the same amount as someone who lives in the
country, there will be a 25 percent greater chance of mortality from lung cancer than if you live in the country, Dr. Epstein said.

The cries of industry that animal testing does not reflect a
true picture of what might happen to the human consumer
do not stand up under Dr. Epstein's scrutiny. He pointed out
that sometimes man is more sensitive, sometimes less, to the
dangers inherent in any given chemical. Echoing back to the
benchmark thalidomide tragedy, he pointed out that women
are 60 times more sensitive to the drug than mice, 100 times
more sensitive than rats, 200 times more sensitive than dogs,
and 700 times more sensitive than hamsters. Facts like these
indicate the critically important role the Delaney amendment plays in protecting the consumer—and the importance
of protecting the amendment from the onslaughts of industry
and some of the high-placed government officials who would
do away with it.

Dr. Epstein, along with many others, had little regard for
the FDA's reliance on cattlemen to assure the consumer that
there would be no stilbestrol remaining in the meat after
slaughter, since only some 500 were tested or sampled out of
30,000,000 cattle produced in 1970. With Sweden banning
U.S. beef unless it is specifically certified by the U.S. Department of Agriculture as additive-free, the question naturally

arises as to why the U.S. consumer should be less protected. And the question remained unanswered.

Senator Ribicoff, taking this situation into consideration and combining it with previous atttudes of the USDA as far as defective meats were concerned, said: "It would seem consistently that the Department of Agriculture, through various administrations, has been careless, negligent, and indifferent to the well-being of the American people."

The tricky question of nitrates and nitrites as additives emerged from the hearings, and the use of these chemicals still poses a very real problem. Nitrites are important in that they can check botulism, which is a very deadly and often fatal form of food poisoning. Nitrites are permitted as food additives in meat and fish at levels of 200 parts per million. The problem comes in when they combine with secondary amines to produce nitrosamines. These in turn can produce cancer and birth defects through the absorption of very small doses. The evidence for this is heavily documented in laboratory tests throughout the world.

Experts like Dr. Epstein are highly suspicious of the use of nitrites at the 200-parts-per-million level, not because of the danger of acute toxicity, but because of the danger of creating intolerable levels of nitrosamines after the chemical has entered the human system. High on the priority list, from Dr. Epstein's point of view, is the urgent necessity to reduce the tolerance of nitrites from 200 parts per million down to a maximum of 20 parts per million. Further, there is a critical need to look for less hazardous alternatives to this preservative.

The difficulty of the situation arises when a conscientious housewife might want to avoid such additives as nitrites or stilbestrol. There are no labeling requirements whatever, and there is no way for the housewife to tell if her food is saturated with these. This situation is compounded by the food manufacturers who insist on the right to determine on their own whether or not a food chemical is safe. Not even the FDA can know under these conditions, let alone the housewife. Flavoring agents, supposed to number around 200, have been used in food without any independent scientific review.

One knotty question involving the whole status of the GRAS list is: Does each item on it serve a generally socially useful purpose? Dr. Epstein's stand was that most of the 600-odd chemicals on the GRAS list would disappear from view if this question were conscientiously applied.

In following this up at the hearings, Senator Ribicoff asked: "In other words, what you are saying is, we are spending millions and millions of dollars for which the consumer ultimately pays for substances which have no basic efficacy?"

"This is my view," Dr. Epstein replied. "But more importantly than my view, sir, there is the fact that there is no requirement for demonstration of efficacy for any area except for drugs. For drugs there is a clear requirement for efficacy, but not for food additives."

Near the end of Dr. Epstein's testimony, Senator Ribicoff asked: "Is there any reasonable and practical way that you and I or our families or every consumer can avoid these harmful and dangerous chemicals in our foods? Or do we just have to take them every time we go to the market?"

Said Dr. Epstein in reply: "This is the great tragedy of the situation. . . . When it comes to food, we have basically no option available to us. You go to the supermarket, you buy processed meat; you have no idea whether there are any nitrites in it. When you buy beef you have no idea whether there are carcinogenic synthetic estrogens in it. We have no choice. Clearly, there have to be requirements for efficacy. . . . Without independent and nonprofit evaluation I would say that you and I are completely impotent. We have no choice."

Arising out of the testimony of the hearings was the inevitable question as to why FDA Commissioner Edwards had not seen fit to follow the advice of three different expert committees (later, there were four). They unanimously recommended that all food chemicals face obligatory testing for their capacity to produce birth defects or gene damage before being put on the market.

The consensus of several scientists is that plans to put these recommendations into action could have begun overnight, even though the facilities for testing might have taken several months to set up. However, nothing was done, and the recommendations merely sat in limbo. Meanwhile, the consumer goes to the supermarket to select bright, fresh red meat cuts jammed with high levels of nitrites principally for the cosmetic purpose of making the meat look good. Or choosing bright orange-color oranges loaded with cosmetic coloring that carries with it a threat to his health. As Senator Charles Percy, on the same subcommittee, put it: "The consumer has faith in his government, that he is buying something that is what it is represented to be—pure food. And we find that the maker is adding more cost to the consumer to put something in the food that adds cost to the product. I think it is the responsibility of government to call them before us to find out why they are doing this. . . ."

The color additive question rose into special importance a few months after the Ribicoff hearings. In the fall of 1971, new Soviet studies revealed that Red No. 2 had been found to prevent pregnancies and create stillbirths in a series of tests on rats. This artificial color had been long in contention.

The FDA sluggishly ordered animal tests to be made on Red No. 2 after the Soviet studies and at the same time instructed food processors using the color to submit lists of all products on which the color is used. In addition, the same type of tests were ordered on other food colorings "to show whether the color additive produces any adverse effects on reproduction." Meanwhile, the FDA's own tests were a year behind the Russians', and its faltering, weak proposals were acknowledged to be the result of the agency's inability to confirm the Russian tests immediately.

Considering the fact that food colors had been under suspicion since the mid-1800's, the FDA's inaction in clarifying this threat has been roundly criticized. The first organic aniline dye was synthesized by William Henry Perkin in 1858, creating the coal-tar dye industry. These dyes were supposed to bring the consumer relief from the poisonous mineral pigments of lead, arsenic, copper, and chromium that were poured into bonbons and candies a century or so ago. When workers in the German dye industry began toppling with a wide spectrum of illnesses, the 1907 Federal Food and Drugs Act began to certify those coal-tar dyes that were supposed to be safe for foods. But even this crude safety system was voluntary, and it wasn't until 1938 when this color certification system was written into the law.

In the 1950's, two separate batches of children came down with severe poisonings from Halloween candy and popcorn soaked with highly concentrated food coloring, principally citrus red 2. This in turn led to the Color Additive Amendments of 1960, calling for the retesting of all food colors.

The Russian tests of 1971, and others like them, indicate that the problem is far from being settled. When the Color Additive Amendments were passed, the same old story popped up again: Delays and stalling prevented them from being put into action for a decade. In the mid-sixties, the FDA announced that it was going to take red 4 off the market, but the maraschino cherry manufacturers outtalked the FDA, which permitted the coloring to remain.

But, again, no scientist living knows what the cumulative effect of the food additive revolution will be. With the advent of the new wave of processed and convenience foods, the problems are multiplying out of hand. (In 1969 processed foods outsold unprocessed ones for the first time.) As Jim Turner put it: "The chemical problems of the 1950's and 1960's are a picnic compared to the problems now developing." He quoted two California doctors, whose study revealed that the practical applicability of the present-day knowledge concerning food additives should alert all doctors to the potential hazards of these agents. They noted that an increasing number of patients have been observed in clinical practice with diffuse hair fall, chronic urticaria (red, patched skin), toxic epidermal, spotted skin, and other newly emerging illnesses. They concluded: "It is common practice to consign these diseases to causes unknown or to classify them as idiosyncratic."

Dr. William Lijinsky, of the University of Nebraska, announced that he was particularly concerned about the excess use of nitrites as color agents, rather than their more restrictive use as preservatives. He indicated that nitrites might contribute significantly to the incidence of lung cancer in cigarette smokers and increase the chances of cancer with consumption of beer, wine, cereals, and certain drugs. (The latter include Ritalin, for overactive children, and Preludin, along with other appetite suppressants—as well as antihistamines.) By using nitrites as preservatives only and not as meat cosmetics, the permitted levels could be reduced by 90 to 95 percent, he argued. Dr. Lijinsky's studies are being carried out under a National Cancer Institute grant.

The guts of the problem seems to lie in the difference between the total freewheeling use of food additives, which the food manufacturers would like to have, or the use of them only under the conditions of a question Senator Percy asked: "Does the chemical in question serve a socially and economically useful purpose for the general population?"

Under this proliferation of food additives, and because scientists admit they cannot possibly assess the potential harm of the more than 3,000 micro-insults the additives bring with them, it would almost seem that the question would answer itself. Legislation is obviously needed to require additives to be effective as well as safe, just as drugs are. The ratio of intake between food and drugs is staggering, even though drugs may be more concentrated. Everybody eats food every day; not everybody takes drugs every day. Why shouldn't the burden of the proof be on the manufacturer to prove this key point before being permitted to use any additive? Until this kind of legislation is put through, consumers continue as a giant group of guinea pigs, and there is little or nothing they can do about it.

Senator Percy singled out the dominating reason for the position of the consumer today: "All of us having young people are impressed with the fact that they are going back and making their own bread. My breakfast cereal that I had this morning, that I have been having for months, is fixed by my own daughter. She won't buy packaged products anymore. She is going to grow her own vegetables. She does not want them contaminated with chemicals. This is not just one daughter—these are hundreds of young people fed up with artificial additions made in food products which are injurious and harmful and expensive."

Every time the food scene is surveyed and summarized by a Congressional hearing, facts emerge that are alarming as far as the consumer is concerned. The comfort that some manufacturers take in the assumption that all chemicals would produce cancer if administered in large enough doses is further refuted by Dr. Umberto Saffiotti, the cancer specialist for the National Cancer Institute. He stated: "We find that only a fraction, only a relatively small percentage of those tested do in fact produce cancers, whereas many others do not." He went on to say that he was surprised that Dr. G. T. Bryan's findings about the cancer-producing qualities of saccharin were not widely publicized in the press. Speaking of this and another study regarding pesticides, he said: "It is a very interesting phenomenon. We would have thought that the lay press would jump on the final documented paper with all the data in it and make news out of it. It did not." Since it didn't, most of the public remains in the dark about this, and saccharin remains on the shelf in millions of bottles of soft drinks and millions of cans of food.

The concern regarding unlabeled caffeine in soft drinks is continually popping up in the testimony of various scientists, especially its effect on children. Sodium bisulphite, used as a preservative in dried fruits—prunes, apricots, raisins, for instance—was pointed out by Dr. Lawrence Fishbein, of the National Institute for Environmental Health Sciences, as being a mutagen hazard. Some scientists have expressed the fear that the largely untested mutagenetic qualities of food additives may be even a greater risk than that of cancer. It is ironic to note that little or none of this questioning comes from industrial scientists or the laboratories they use to check out the industry-inspired additives. It is the common consensus in the food field that a laboratory which gets a reputation for turning down chemicals as dangerous soon finds itself without any industrial clients.

At the present time there is no micrometer built to measure accurately the danger of the micro-insults we're all exposed to. An innocent chemical outside the body might turn to a demon once it is swallowed. There is little the concerned public can do at the moment, except to support consumer organizations and members of Congress who are willing to take vigorous, active stands against the abuses of industry and the lassitude of FDA policy makers who persistently are inclined to hold hands with the men they are supposed to regulate.

11

Of Poisons and Death

SAMUEL COCHRAN, Jr., of Bedford Village, New York, had everything to live for. He was a vice-president of the Bank of New York on Fifth Avenue and had a lovely home and family. On the evening of June 29, 1971, he and his wife sat down to dinner, and each of them took only a sip or two of some chilled Bon Vivant vichyssoise. It tasted so bad, they couldn't finish it.

On his commuter train to Grand Central Station the next morning, Mr. Cochran began to notice that his eyes were not acting at all normally. His vision was blurred, and he was seeing double. By noon the condition worsened, and he was able to set an appointment with Dr. Richard Darrell, an eye specialist, in the early afternoon. By the time his examination was finished, it was obvious to the specialist that there was more to this than eye trouble. There was a distinct possibility of a stroke, and Dr. Darrell immediately arranged for Mr. Cochran to see his family doctor and for Mrs. Cochran to drive in to pick him up.

By 4:30 that afternoon, he was back in the suburbs for an examination by Dr. Henry Colmore, who had been the family's physician for over twenty years.

The symptoms were perplexing. Mr. Cochran's tongue was thick, his arms were weak and trembling, he was still seeing double. He could not talk or swallow. By the time he was taken to the Northern Westchester Hospital for consultation with a neurologist, it was obvious that his cranial nerves were failing rapidly. But, strangely enough, his knee-jerk reflexes were perfectly normal.

Although the stroke diagnosis seemed unlikely, an anticoagulant was prescribed. In midevening, a report from the hospital indicated that Mr. Cochran's condition was satisfactory, and Dr. Colmore went to bed.

Shortly after eleven that night, the hospital called Dr. Colmore to tell him that Mr. Cochran was dead. The paralysis had moved from his tongue to his throat to his lungs, and he simply stopped breathing. Dr. Colmore notified Mrs. Cochran, who in turn called her two sons. They drove up from New York City to join her in her bereavement.

But in the early hours of the morning, Dr. Colmore was again awakened. This time it was a call from the Cochran sons, who advised him that their mother was seriously ill. Her speech, too, was thick and labored. It was obviously more, much more, than grief and hysteria over her husband's death. She began duplicating all of the other symptoms her husband had suffered.

At this point, something jelled in Dr. Colmore's mind. The rare disease that the vast majority of doctors never encounter in their entire careers suddenly seemed to be the only answer: botulism. It is the most deadly form of food poisoning known. It is said authoritatively that a few thimbles of the toxin produced by the botulinus bacteria could wipe out everybody on earth.

When Mrs. Cochran mentioned the vichyssoise she and her husband had the night before, Dr. Colmore was almost certain. She was rushed to a New York hospital for intensive care.

The empty, discarded can was found. It was also taken to the hospital for analysis. Meanwhile, public health officials were notified, and one of the most massive food recalls in FDA history began.

Botulism is the disease caused by the bacteria known as *C. botulinum*. These are spore-forming microorganisms that can be found in both the soil and water of many different areas of the country. The spores themselves are not harmful. A considerable number of raw fruits and vegetables bear them. But under certain conditions, the botulinus bacteria can grow from the spores and produce the deadly toxin that causes the disease. Over the last ten years, there have fortunately been only fifty deaths from it. Twenty-four of these happened in 1963, a year when seven persons died from eating smoked whitefish and chubs processed in the Great Lakes area. The reason: inadequate heating, which failed to kill the bacteria. An absolute must in treating susceptible foods to prevent botulism is that they must be heated for at least thirty minutes at 240° F.

Botulinum cannot grow in the presence of oxygen. Because of this, canned foods are the most frequent carriers of the lethal toxin when they are inadequately heated after canning. But frozen, precooked foods can be guilty if they are held at temperatures permitting growth. Home canning is most often recorded as the cause of botulism deaths, but it is the commercially canned foods that are most dangerous because of their widespread distribution. Food preparation in the current era is centralized. Mass distribution is rapid. Consequently, a mass outbreak can happen almost overnight. In 1970, some 80,000 pizzas of the Roman Inn Pizza Company in Eau Claire, Wisconsin, flooded the market from the Dakotas to western Pennsylvania and New York. Small bits of mushrooms sprinkled as topping on the pizzas were found to contain botulinum B, one of several types of the bacteria. Warnings were rushed out by the FDA to homes, restaurants, pizza parlors, and institutions, and the company cooperated in recalling the suspect pizzas.

But this was microscopic compared to the recall of the Bon Vivant products, including not only vichyssoise but the seventy other products produced by the company.

While Mrs. Cochran remained in critical condition, treated with a special botulism antitoxin and aided by a mechanical respirator, the staggering job of pulling back nearly 1,000,000 cans of Bon Vivant products began. Complicating the procedure, and making it almost impossible for a consumer to be selective in the types of soup she might be buying, was that Bon Vivant packed soup for over a score of other distributors under their own labels. These included several impressive carriage-trade companies: Gristedes, Marshall Field, S. S. Pierce, and others. A consumer, even if warned, would have to memorize a list of products that went on to include Braden's, Wolferman's, S & W Fine Foods, Honey Bear Farms, Thalheimer's, White Rose, Connoisseur, Penn Dutch, Monarch, Hickory Farms, and still others. There was nothing on these labels to indicate that these soups or products had been packed by the Bon Vivant company, so that a housewife might easily pick up one of these cans confident that she was protecting her family from the suspect shipments of Bon Vivant.

It is a tribute to the FDA and local health authorities that only one known death was traced to the lethal vichyssoise. Once the presence of *C. botulinum* was confirmed, warnings and seizures went into action. Vichyssoise, cold leek-and-potato soup of elegance, became a word that sent shudders through consumers. There were approximately 6,500 cans of lot V-141 (so labeled because it was made on May 21, the 141st day of the year, with the initial *V* standing for the type of soup). Four cans were found in the same store in Katonah, New York, where Mrs. Cochran had bought the groceries for the tragic meal.

Three of these were swollen—a typical symptom of the possibility of botulinum within a can. Andrew Paretti, the distressed president of the company, cooperated fully in the recall. A mouse injected with the soup died within twenty-four hours. Four more cans of lot V-141 tested were found to be contaminated, as the giant collection job continued among some 28,000 wholesalers and retailers. But twenty days after the tragedy, almost 2,000 cans of the suspect V-141 lot were still missing.

FDA inspectors looked for—and found—cans that hinted at trouble within. These included *springers,* where if an end of the can is pressed, it will move in and out; *flippers,* where if one end is pushed, the other end moves out; *leakers,* where substance is actually leaking from the can; and soft or hard *swells,* where the can is swollen so that it can be pressed in or not, depending on the "hardness." Deeply dented cans, where the seam might have sprung or the enamel within the can cracked also came under suspicion, along with rust spots.

But since contamination cannot always be smelled or tasted, only the painstaking laboratory tests would be able to tell the whole story. Samples of each can were prepared for injection into mice for testing.

Meanwhile, attention was turned to determining the how and why of the tragedy. Bon Vivant, Inc., had been in business since 1863. Although its sales totaled some 4,000,000 cans of various soups and sauces a year, it was not a large plant, employing about fifty people. It was obvious that something was wrong with the plant's quality control. In April and May, the company's canning equipment had to be repaired five times. New findings revealed that underprocessing was evident in at least six other codes of Bon Vivant soups, whether under its own label or among the private brands that the company packed, including its black bean soup. From Kansas City, the report came that abnormalities were evident in several cans of other Bon Vivant soups, in addition to the vichyssoise. An international warning was sent out to foreign customers, and the FDA's interstate travel sanitation branch warned airline caterers that might be using the soup.

The FDA investigation ultimately produced evidence to show that the company failed to heat the soup to the proper temperature of 240° F for the minimum thirty-minute time span after sealing. Pointing up the manpower problems that the FDA continually faces, the Bon Vivant plant had not been inspected for over four years. With only thirty inspectors to cover the entire state of New Jersey, it is almost impossible for the consumer to be properly protected.

Unfortunately, the problem is not confined to the Bon Vivant incident. Not too long after the search for the canned soups sprawled around the country, the Campbell Soup Company discovered the deadly botulinus bacteria in a large batch of its chicken-vegetable soup produced at a Texas plant. Again another frenzied search and recall was conducted. This time there were no reported deaths, but again the thin resources of the FDA were stretched to combat a potentially dangerous problem.

At just about the same time that the Bon Vivant crisis was taking place, another major contamination incident erupted. The discovery began at Holly Farms of Wilkesboro, North Carolina, when Dr. Kenneth May, director of research and quality control, began to notice that chickens at what is believed to be the world's largest producer of broilers were experiencing an extremely low rate of hatching. He began running tests on the feed that the chickens were given and discovered that the fish meal that made up a considerable portion of the feed was contaminated with PCB. This is an extremely toxic chemical that is known to cause gastric distress in humans and birth defects and liver damage to laboratory animals. Its full effect on humans has never been tested. Seven federal agencies were suddenly and dramatically called into action to survey the chemical in the fall of 1971, when it was realized that extensive industrial use of this could have farther-reaching effects than those of DDT.

PCB is very similar to DDT in that it remains intact in nature and builds up cumulatively. Dr. May contacted Monsanto Chemical, the exclusive manufacturer of PCB, and with the help of the FDA and the Department of Agriculture, the source was tracked down to the East Coast Terminal, Wilmington, North Carolina. Over a four-month period the chemical had leaked from machinery onto some 16,000 tons of fish meal being prepared for chicken feed which was widely distributed in many parts of the country. Again a search was begun, because millions of chickens fed with the contaminated product were already on the market, and it was impossible to predict how many others would be. Holly Farms alone destroyed 77,000 chickens. The full extent of the damage has never been accurately assessed. Meanwhile, an uncounted number of consumers were exposed to a potentially dangerous risk.

But the chain of events didn't stop there. Over 400,000 eggs were similarly contaminated from the same substance in the process, and ineffective attempts were made by the FDA to clear them from the market. One shipment of 168,000 to Washington and another of 14,000 were supposed to have been seized on arrival. But when FDA officials arrived to do so, they found nothing to seize. Jack Walden, the FDA's press relations chief, indicated that he had to assume the eggs had arrived and had already been sold to consumers. "I guess we missed them," he said.

A whole new story on PCB is just beginning to develop. FDA officials appear confused and flustered about it. Monsanto Chemical, the principal producer of the chemical, is tight-lipped. Britain has banned the chemical altogether. At least five have died from cooking oil contaminated with it in Japan. It has been found imbedded in cereal boxes and widely used in various industrial processes. It has killed thousands of fish and marine birds.

Meanwhile, and again roughly during the same time period, eleven persons were stricken with a staphylococcus infection from eating some of Hormel's vacuum-packed Genoa salami, and nine persons came down with the same infection from a similar product made by the Armour Company. Only a few months before all this, World's Finest Candies, known for its sales to civic groups and charitable organizations for fund-raising purposes, discovered that a large batch of chocolate candy and cake frosting was riddled with salmonella organisms, one of the widest-spread causes of all food-borne diseases. Although it is not as deadly as botulism, its frequency and prevalence make it a larger threat to the consumer. And it can be fatal.

There are over 1,000 different strains of the bacteria, named after Dr. D. E. Salmon who isolated the first strain of this group in 1885. No one knows how many people come down with it each year in the United States. One educated guess is 2,000,000. Others believe that this figure is too low. With the advent of the large processors performing as giant community kitchens, some scientists feel that the chances for wider epidemics are increasing, moving from the Sunday school picnic outbreaks into large interstate epidemics.

There are other reasons why chances for more severe outbreaks have increased. People are eating out more, in schools, restaurants, and factories. Consumption has increased in raw or slightly heated meats and poultry. Mass production of processed foods has increased. It is becoming recognized that more foods and even medicines are capable of carrying salmonella. Dried milk, smoked fish, and yeast have been added to the long list that is salmonella-prone. Cats, dogs, and other pets have been pinpointed as culprits, along with the stale portions of pet food they are likely to leave in their dishes.

Follow-up studies on some salmonella outbreaks have shown the number of reported cases to be vastly underestimated. In Riverside, California, 200 cases were reported. Epidemiologists rechecked the area to find that 16,000 was the more accurate figure. In Oxford, Nebraska, 5 persons were reported to come down with gastroenteritis after eating contaminated turkeys. A follow-up stool survey showed that at least 261 were infected.

The salmonella bacteria grow swiftly in the gastrointestinal tract when they are taken into the body. Nausea, vomiting, abdominal cramps, diarrhea, and fever often follow. Infants and the elderly are hit worst, along with invalids of any age. The bacteria grow markedly in certain foods when they are left even briefly at room temperature.

Infection comes often from the silent carriers—food handlers who themselves show no signs of the disease. Workers in abattoirs frequently bring the disease home. Even babies are guilty. They can harbor the infection for longer periods than adults. Mechanical agents for carrying the disease beside food can include toys, towels, toilet seats, and pets. Young turtles sold as pets are particularly liable to be carriers, because they are often hatched and raised in severely contaminated ponds. In the retail stores where the turtles are sold, the conditions under which they are kept are seldom sanitary. Dried flies and insects fed to the turtles don't enhance these conditions.

Eggs and egg products are high on the list of salmonella-carrying foods. Grade A eggs without cracks are seldom guilty, but bread and cake mixes can easily be infected by one egg. Fresh pork sausages have often been found to be contaminated. One survey in Florida showed the rate of contamination to be 8 percent in the product of national processors and up to 58 percent for those from local abbatoirs.

The problem with salmonella in poultry has been increased with the advent of partially cooked or ready-to-eat poultry products. The importance of pasteurization of milk and cheese is demonstrated by the prevalence of salmonella in unpasteurized products. Among other sources of the infection that have been incriminated from time to time are dried yeast, dried cereal, dried coconut, sauces and salad dressings, bakery products, cream-filled desserts and toppings, gelatin, synthetic ice cream, pickles, and various kinds of sandwiches prepared for vending machines. Lettuce contaminated by the drippings from a frozen chicken was responsible for one salmonellosis outbreak.

The leftovers in pet food dishes are dangerous, because they are often left there for many hours. When time comes to wash the dish out, it is done halfheartedly. With the increase in the preparation of food in retail outlets, new dangers have emerged. One outbreak in the Pacific Northwest revealed that barbecued chickens were not properly stored after cooking. Allowing food to remain at room temperature for any length of time can be dangerous. Trouble begins at about 45° F and continues up to about 113° F, with about 100° as the ideal temperature for the salmonella bacteria to grow and flourish. Even with this in mind, salmonellae can remain very much alive in frozen foods. Some survived on poultry carcasses that had been quick frozen at −35° F and kept frozen for over a year. If it's any comfort, acid vegetables and fruits show little danger of containing the bacteria.

The FDA has set down some suggestions to housewives

about the threat of this widespread infection, which include thorough washing of foods and hands, careful following of instructions on labels, thorough cooking, and prompt refrigeration in the kitchen or especially on picnics.

A United Nations food committee recently expressed its concern about the whole problem of contamination of foods throughout the world. In one of its reports, it said:

> Salmonellosis seems to be increasing in a number of countries. Food poisoning outbreaks due to Staphylococcus enterotoxin and to Clostridium perfringens remain common. Deaths from botulism still occur. . . . Contemporary trends in processing technology demonstrate a much increased need for microbiological examination of foods as a means of assessing safety. The hazard of food poisoning is otherwise likely to increase as new foods or foods prepared and packaged by modified methods are marketed in ever increasing quantities without adequate investigation of the selective effect of the introduced changes upon the microbial ecology of foods. The efficiency of modern marketing may accentuate the risk for, should a consignment of food be significantly contaminated, widespread disease could result before effective recall of the food would be practicable.

Other comments on the contamination food front are not at all cheerful. R. Paul Elliot, the FDA's microbiology coordinator, in a comment for a food and drug officials' symposium, began his remarks with: "How much do we know of the incidence of food-borne disease in this country? Far too little!" Like other experts, he was particularly concerned with the more than two billion pounds of convenience foods Americans consume every year. He emphasized the importance of never keeping precooked foods out for more than an hour or so between the temperatures of 40° F and 120° F. This sort of violation is most likely to occur in the hands of consumers, he noted. Products that undergo less severe processing techniques, such as pasteurized canned hams and pasteurized chicken or crabmeat, are also hazardous if they are subjected to room temperatures for any length of time. Chilled but above-freezing temperatures can, however, be protective for some time. The problem is that mildly heat-processed foods are increasing in variety and quantity, including poultry, meat products, and party dips. He pointed out that while the automatic vending machines are designed to hold foods below 50° F, some bacteria can grow heartily at about 45° F. Food-handling machinery, he noted, is designed for production efficiency that brings profits—often neglecting microbial problems. Catered meals, commissary foods, salads, and cream- or custard-filled bakery goods are often at the bottom of food poisoning outbreaks and bear special scrutiny.

One of the big problems is that a low bacterial count for a raw food product is meaningful, but in a processed food it does not necessarily guarantee safety, according to E. M. Foster, professor of bacteriology at the University of Wisconsin. In one case, the bacterial count on a batch of dried milk gave no indication of abnormality. But serious staphylococcal poisoning resulted from it. The reason: The original whole milk had been held for several hours without proper refrigeration before drying. Staphylococci grew in the milk and produced the toxin that creates the poisoning. When the product went through the preheating and drying process, the bacteria were killed but the toxin remained, unobserved by microscopic examination.

Sometimes the processing that kills off those organisms that produce decay and other obvious signs of food spoilage simply permits more dangerous toxins to grow that provide no warning to the consumer. A housewife will throw away a bad-smelling fish, but if a processor is more intent on keeping his product salable than in keeping it safe, there is danger in the wind. The basic problem with frozen, precooked, ready-to-eat products is that they are merely thawed and warmed by the housewife. If the processor has slipped up on adequate heating or permitted prolonged holding before freezing, or if the product has been thawed and refrozen, a clear hazard exists. There is no question that fresh food, thoroughly cooked, is the safest.

Staphylococci infection, more often referred to as staph,

ranks along with salmonellosis and botulism as a potent consumer hazard. The bacteria are small and sphere-shaped
and sometimes gather in clusters, like grapes. The poisonings
from its toxins rank along with salmonellosis in prevalence.
More often than not, the staph germ gets into foods through
infected persons who handle it. The bacteria thrive on the
hands and arms, in the nose and hair. Symptoms are similar
to salmonellosis and usually appear within three to eight
hours after consumption. Housewives would do well to ob-
serve strict personal cleanliness in the kitchen, as well as
storing foods under refrigeration and cooking thoroughly.

Other hazards that plague the consumer are shigella, the
rod-shaped bacteria that comes from the intestines of man,
and *Clostridium perfringens.* This also is found in the intestines
of man, in addition to soil and dust. Like botulinum, this
rod-shaped bacterium cannot grow in air. *E. coli* bacteria are
also dangerous, because they indicate contamination with
fecal material. Nearly all the general rules of caution apply
in combating these. In the prevention of *perfringens* contamination, experts suggest that meats should be held hot and
served hot, that leftovers should be cooled rapidly in small
lots, and that leftover meats should be well heated before re-
serving. Leftover gravy should be brought to a rolling boil.
Cold cuts should be maintained cold and served cold—not at
room temperature.

The Bon Vivant crisis brought with it many questions that
the consumer is prompted to ask about canned foods, as well
as the whole picture on food poisoning in the modern age. If
canned foods are kept in a dry place at moderate temperatures, they will keep indefinitely as long as the container
doesn't leak. One year maximum, however, is recommended.
A single freezing and thawing of a can is usually harmless,
although the ends of the can should return to a normal flat-
ness after thawing. Foods can be kept in an open can in the
refrigerator, although acid foods should be moved to glass
jars because they have a tendency to dissolve some of the iron
in the can. The stains you see on the inside of an otherwise
sound can are not harmful, but rust on the outside of a can is

a spoilage warning. Further, the FDA warns, if the ends bulge, or if the contents have an abnormal odor or appearance, throw the can away without tasting the contents at all. One lick of the contents of a botulinum-riddled can could be fatal.

Contrary to the food additive picture, the dangers from food contamination are shared equally by both the processor and the consumer. The hazards are many, but at least the consumer can be sure that this is one area where the manufacturer is as anxious as the consumer to avoid them. And a strong motivation for the manufacturer to avoid contamination is clearly obvious: Food poisoning is downright unprofitable; additives are not.

12

On the Wings of Mercury
and Pesticides

THE CARTOON in *The New Yorker* was deceivingly simple. It showed a huge factory on the bank of a river. There was a high stone abutment, rising from the river to a terrace by the factory. There were several huge sewage pipes spewing out liquids into the river with enormous force. There were two men—it was easy to extrapolate that they were environmental officers of some sort—plus an archetype of a factory owner between them. All three were looking down at the sewage pipes. The factory owner was surprised, and the caption had him saying: "So *that's* where it goes! Well, I'd like to thank you fellows for bringing it to my attention."

The cartoon crystallized in a few brief strokes of the pen the entire guts of the enormously threatening pollution problem. Its incisive interpretation of the truth cannot be challenged. For thousands of factories all over the country are doing exactly this same thing, and the owners or managers or directors are constantly saying: "We have never knowingly created pollution."

In no place is this more evident than in the mercury story —a modern ghost and horror story of the corporation soul.

Mercury, along with the other intentional and unintentional poisons in our food, is a silent, undetectable ghost—a ghost we can't see, can't taste, can't touch without sophisticated scientific instruments. Yet it, along with other indirect hazards such as pesticides, herbicides, and animal feed, adds to our intolerable burden of micro-insults. The end result is a growing burden that baffles science and boggles the mind.

The mercury story began quietly, insidiously, and not recently, as many people think.

Even in the unenlightened days of 1673, the Austrian government stepped in to limit the time spent by mercury miners to four hours a day and no more than eight days in a month. The mercury vapor that they inhaled was taking a tremendous toll of lives.

The "mad hatter" story was, of course, well-known in the days of the Industrial Revolution, the "madness" being caused by the mercury fumes created by the production of felt. Hat workers would go inexplicably mad and die.

Environmental mercury began to show itself with a vengeance in 1953. Minamata, Japan, rests on a bay of the same name, and local fishermen were proud of their catches in it. But some of them began coming down with strange symptoms, and as others joined them, the disease reached epidemic proportions by 1956. Over 100 persons faced the agonizing symptoms of the poisoning: the blurred vision, the sleeplessness, the constant trembling, the loss of weight, the drunkenlike staggering—and for many, death. Nearly 60 of the fishermen and members of their families died.

Some 19 congenital cases of brain-damaged children were born to mothers whose diet consisted mainly of seafood. Other congenital neurological injuries were well documented, demonstrating how easily methyl mercury can slip through the placental barrier. A very curious result was noted: In many cases, the mothers showed no mercury poisoning symptoms at all. Only the deformed children bore the brunt of the disease, indicating that the fetus was more sensitive than the mother.

But where was the mercury coming from?

On the shores of Minamata Bay was a chemical plant. Using a large volume of mercury as a catalyst, it had been gushing out its wastes into the bay, depositing large amounts of the chemical that were assumed to fall to the bottom and never rise again. Mercury is over thirty times heavier than water.

But then it became apparent that something else was happening. The pure element mercury is a metal, and while it's nothing you'd want to sprinkle over your dessert, it is ten times less toxic than the organic form of mercury known as methyl mercury. It became apparent that the Japanese fishermen had died from the organic form of the metal, while the factory was spilling out the other form. How could this happen?

The answer lay in the bacteria on the bottom of the bay. They could work on the metal lying in the sludge on the bottom which, especially if it is oily, can act as a reservoir building up large deposits of methyl mercury. This, in turn, could be freed and rise from the bottom to contaminate both the fish and the water. In the Minamata area, the fish contained large amounts of the deadly organic methyl mercury. This sort of compound is very slowly metabolized in animals and builds up in the tissues. In foodstuffs, this is critically dangerous.

Little was heard about the Minamata disaster in 1956, in spite of the fact that it foreshadowed a growing potential disaster. And very little interest was aroused when a similar mercury incident took place in Iraq in 1961. Within a year, the scene shifted back to Japan, to the city of Niigata. Here the victims were again fishermen, here the poisons were traced to another industrial plant, and here 30 persons were stricken. Six of them died.

During this period, concern was growing in Sweden over methyl mercury seed dressings, which had been used as fungicides since the 1940's. Seed-eating birds were felled in droves from the mercury they consumed. Swedish scientists also began to notice the crops even with small amounts of methyl mercury brought serious problems up the food chain, either when man ate the crop directly or ingested the methyl mercury indirectly by eating animals that had fed on the affected crops. By 1965 Swedish officials clamped down on the use of mercury seed dressings, and the mercury content of foods dropped with the action.

Two years after this, Sweden again had a mercury problem. Fish began showing up with large concentrations of mercury compounds. Again, the pollution was traced to factories. One source was the pulp and paper factories. Another source was factories that produced caustic soda and chlorine, known as chlor-alkali plants. Fish from designated waters in Sweden were declared unfit for human consumption.

The situation was so alarming to the Swedes that in 1966—four years before any action was taken in the United States—they held an international conference on the mercury problem. Five U.S. government scientists were in attendance. At the conference, the picture that emerged was exactly the same as we have seen today. The pattern of the current mercury problem was predicted in detail. The information developed at the conference was inescapable. But nothing happened.

While Sweden was taking action, the U.S. Public Health Service, a department of HEW, was surveying the waters of the Detroit River on the Michigan side of Lake Erie. The agency completed a long and exhaustive report on the pollution of the waters. Not one mention of mercury was made in it.

An ominous note was struck in 1969. One evening, Ernest Huckleby, of Alamogordo, New Mexico, accidentally poured out for his hogs a batch of grain that had been dressed with a methyl mercury fungicide. After the hogs had been slaughtered and eaten, tragedy struck the family. Three of his children came down with frightening symptoms. One of them found it impossible to speak. Another went blind. A third went into a deep coma. All are still irreparably damaged. The source: mercury residues in the meat of the hogs they had eaten. The villain: Panogen, a mercury-based fungicide. It is still permitted in the United States, although Sweden stopped production on the grounds that it would be immoral to export a product that was banned at home.

The sophisticated scientific communication channels we

possess in this modern age were simply not functioning. The caustic soda-chlorine plants in North America continued pumping out mercury-laden wastes, to the tune of as high as 200 pounds a day from the Ontario Dow Chemical plant into the St. Clair River. The chlor-alkali industry, as it is called, has been throwing out about 400 tons of the element into the environment each year. In the St. Clair River, the mercury concentration in the sludge is approaching the yield of 4 pounds of mercury per ton, which is just about the same concentration the commercial operators find profitable to mine.

In May, 1969, a lead article in the magazine *Environment* came out with a strong story on mercury pollution and its threat. *Nature* had already examined the question less fully about a year before. It would seem most unlikely for major mercury producers to be unaware of such an article appearing in a leading environmental publication. But apparently no one noticed it—or at least never advanced the information that he did. Meanwhile, the offenders, as in the cartoon in *The New Yorker*, continued pouring forth their dubious gift to the public. They included, in addition to Dow, Wyandotte, Du Pont, Allied Chemical, Diamond Shamrock, Georgia Pacific, Olin Mathieson, Weyerhaeuser, B. F. Goodrich, Kaiser, Monsanto, Stauffer Chemical, U.S. Plywood, Shell, Aluminum Corporation of America, Hercules, Scott Paper, and many others—nearly all of them companies that like to noise it about that they are in business for the service of mankind. Major users of the mercury processed in this country include the manufacturers of electrical equipment, chlorine-caustic soda for cleaning and disinfectant agents and for mildew-proofing and agricultural pesticides.

It was strange, in the light of all this activity, especially since 1950, that it took a young Scandinavian graduate student in zoology from the University of Ontario to open up the mercurial Pandora's box.

What he did was very simple. He took a fish from Lake Erie. He tested it. It contained dangerous levels of mercury. He reported it to Canadian officials.

The first time that Ralph Purdy, executive secretary of the
Michigan Water Resources Commission, heard about the situation, he freely admits, was on February 11, 1970. Canadian officials indicated their concern, and Purdy began
checking on the possible sources of mercury contamination.
He found three chlor-alkali plants, but only one of them was
using mercury in the process. It was the Wyandotte Chemical Company. Canada, meanwhile, tracked down major pollution from the Dow Chemical plant at Sarnia, Ontario, on
the melancholy banks of the St. Clair River. But actually,
the Dow plant already had that pointed out by its own waste
control engineer in 1969. Dow claims it began a "crash program" to stop all this stuff in February, 1970, when it ce-
mented shut those big sewer outlets.

Apparently, Dow-Canada wasn't speaking to Dow-U.S.,
or Dow-U.S. wasn't speaking to the FDA or any other government agency, because the first wind the FDA got of the
seriousness of the situation was on March 20, 1970, when the
Canadian Food and Drug Directorate formally advised the
FDA that fish taken from the boundary of Lake St. Clair
contained high mercury residues. The river of the same name
flows into this lake, and this in turn flows into the Detroit
River, then on to Lake Erie, which has long been overbur-
dened with *other* pollutants.

Within a few days, Ontario officials closed the lake to commercial fishing as far as the Canadian waters of both Lake
St. Clair and Lake Erie were concerned. Later, sports fishing
was included in the ban, and the states bordering the waters
established their own bans.

Technically and legally, the limit for mercury residues in
foods of any kind is zero. An interim limit has been set for .5
parts per million by the FDA, but this is ten times more than
the Russians and the World Health Organization suggest as
a guideline. Meanwhile, the junk settles at the bottom of the
rivers, and the corporations report steady profits as they continue on the road to moral bankruptcy.

Said William Glick, vice-president in charge of operation
for the Wyandotte division responsible for the mercury pollu-

tion in Michigan: "Everyone at Wyandotte is extremely concerned that in a few short weeks our reputation of operating responsibly should be damaged by statements and actions that surely have led many people to believe that we have knowingly poisoned public waters with mercury discharges from our plant."

Wyandotte had no permit from the Army Corps of Engineers covering outfall sewers to discharge chemical wastes.

Said C. B. Branch, executive vice-president of Dow Chemical, Midland, Michigan: "We have not knowingly or intentionally contributed to the problem."

The Dow Ontario plant pumped as much as 200 pounds a day into the St. Clair River. Mr. Branch said he first heard about all this mercury fuss when he read about it in the press.

The concentration of 10 parts per million set off the deaths in Minamata in Japan. In the Trenton Channel of the Detroit River, a mile below the Wyandotte Chemical plant outfall, the concentration was found to be 86 parts per million. Sediments below the outfall of General Electric's plant at Edmore, Michigan, in Lake Erie have been found to be 430 parts per million. A similar picture emerges all over the country, wherever mercury is used.

Ralph Nader didn't take kindly to all this. "Why did it take so long for industry and pollution authorities to realize the danger?" he asked. "Companies in the paper, chemical, and plastic industries have known about the dumping of mercury into the waterways or its release into the air." Then he added: "Can the Federal Government afford any longer to spend annually less than one-tenth the cost of a nuclear submarine to test its food products for hazards?"

And then he brought up a very interesting point: If a corporation can be thrown into bankruptcy for not paying its creditors, why shouldn't there be comparable standards for environmental bankruptcy, where a firm displays persistently violent environmental behavior? Are the stakes any lower than nonpayment of company bills?

It is not very cheering to note that the hazards of mercury

are cumulative; they don't fade with time even if the commercial abuses were stopped totally as of this moment. (To say nothing of the long, legal drag-out fights. Allied Chemical, Diamond Shamrock, Olin Mathieson, Oxford Paper, and Weyerhaeuser, among others, were fighting injunctions against their dumpings the moment the crisis broke.) Nor is it equally cheering to learn that there are contaminated rivers in Maine and Georgia, New York, Louisiana, Tennessee, Kentucky, Washington, Delaware, Alabama, Texas, North Carolina, West Virginia, among others, in addition to Michigan and Wisconsin. Over 350 miles of the Wisconsin River shows heavy mercury contamination—*even though the sources of the mercury contamination were closed down in 1958.*

There are other ghosts waiting in the wings to follow mercury. There are disturbing levels of arsenic in many waters, along with other metals. There is a growing problem of lead in oysters. One study has shown lead levels in shellfish of as high as 17 parts per million of lead, 8 parts per million of cadmium, and 4,120 parts per million for zinc.

The widespread problem with mercury in tuna and swordfish is too well known to dwell on in detail here. (Only one cheerful bit of news has appeared recently regarding canned seafood. If you should suddenly find yourself biting on what seems to be glass in your canned tuna or shrimp, the chances are it's a natural crystalline substance known as struvite, which sometimes forms in canned seafood. It's not the most pleasant thing to bite into, but it doesn't affect the safety of the food at all. And it's easy to test whether it's glass or struvite. Drop the substance into some warm vinegar for a while. The struvite will disappear, but the glass will still be around. Unfortunately, the mercury situation is not that easy, and there is no simple test.)

While tuna exceeding the FDA guideline on mercury was found to represent only 3 or 4 percent of the total marketed, the story with swordfish turned out to be a different kettle of fish, because, as a larger fish than tuna, it was farther up the food chain. Finally, in May, 1971, the FDA advised Americans to stop eating swordfish because more than 90 percent of the samples showed excess amounts of mercury.

The mercury—and other heavy-metal—problem is insidious. Most industrial waters are polluted with raw sewage, which speeds up the actions of the microorganisms which change metal mercury into the deadly methyl mercury, ten times as powerful a poison. These mercury compounds are metabolized very slowly and build up in animal and human tissues, striking the brain cells and central nervous system. The main insidious factor is that even if all the sources of mercury pollution are detected and stopped from spilling their wastes in the air and water, the effects on fish will continue for up to 100 years or more. Any attempt to dredge up the poisonous sludge—even if that were physically possible— would simply release the many layers already covered up and could make matters worse. Add to this the cumulative effect of all the other hard and deadly pesticides, plus the estrogens and antibiotics pumped into our foods, and the picture of industrial venality and shortsightedness becomes hideous.

On a recent July morning, a nine-year-old boy by the name of Charles Thomas was playing in a south Jersey tomato field next to the one where his father and brothers and sisters were picking tomatoes. The plants were wet and glistening—but not with morning dew. It was a pesticide residue, sprinkled by airplanes the day before. John Thomas, the father, was a migrant farm worker, facing all the vicissitudes that accompany that sort of job. Suddenly, and without warning, a lumbering, slow-speed airplane swooped down from the sky, and at an altitude so low that a grown adult would run or duck, it began spraying the field with a pesticide. The young boy had no chance to do either. The plane swooped over him, and he was soaked with the spray.

Very shortly, he began to vomit, and his face started swelling. By the next day, the swelling had disappeared, but the father took him to a doctor in Bridgeton, New Jersey, believing that he apparently was suffering from an attack of asthma. Later that day, he seemed to have recovered.

Within two days, however, the swelling returned with a vengeance—this time on his arms, legs, and chest. He was rushed to a hospital in Philadelphia. He died several weeks later, with a working diagnosis of insecticide poisoning.

In Tijuana, Mexico, officials were startled in 1967 when they discovered over 500 people suddenly stricken with severe illnesses. Of these, 16 subsequently died. The cause was finally traced to their eating bread that had been contaminated with the pesticide Parathion.

In the same year, some 1,800 citizens of Qatar and Saudi Arabia were rushed to hospitals after eating bread that had been soaked with an endrin pesticide that had leaked onto flour from two drums in a ship's hold. Twenty-six of the victims died.

A year later, 23 Texas farm workers found themselves seriously ill. The evening before, the cotton field they worked in had been sprayed with Parathion.

The stories are continuous and persistent, from a father who sprinkled an organophosphate insecticide around his house only to poison himself and two children to two babies in St. Louis who died when a disinfectant containing sodium pentacholorophenate was used in washing their diapers.

The whole problem of pesticide residues in both foods and the environment is no less threatening than the mercury crisis. Along with all the other pollution, the country is undergoing what Senator George McGovern calls environmental violence. The industrial polluters have been allowed to continue assaulting the atmosphere as long as they can show some kind of economic benefit. When Congress tries to push through laws that would facilitate the ability of the concerned private citizen to bring legal action against polluters, the National Association of Manufacturers and the U.S. Department of Justice, hand in hand, oppose the action.

Senator Philip Hart of Michigan encountered just such a roadblock in pressing for the Environmental Protection Act of 1970, under which an individual doesn't have to wait for a sluggish Department of Interior or FDA or Department of Agriculture to act. He could, under this bill, get the courts to stop a factory in his town from pouring chemical sewage into his river, for instance.

The Justice Department will tell you, if Shiro Kashiwa, an Assistant Attorney General, is to be believed, that if they prosecute a company causing "unreasonable pollution," it will be "very, very difficult for the government." The officials of the National Association of Manufacturers will say, if their official statement against Senator Hart's bill is to be believed, that the only way to stop pollution is "through cooperation between industrial companies and regulatory officials in working out effective programs based on reasonable time-tables." They say this with a straight face in the light of the whole ugly history of the industrial polluters that are the main core of their membership.

If the Justice Department seems to act as the handmaiden of industry, the United States Department of Agriculture goes right along with it. It is supposed to see to it that the Federal Insecticide, Fungicide, and Rodenticide Act is enforced for the benefit of the consumer. However, for a twenty-year period from 1947 on, the Department of Agriculture's Pesticide Regulation Division failed to recall *any* pesticides that violated the act. Beyond that, over 1,600 different pesticide products were allowed to remain on the market, over the strenuous protests of the HEW. When a product appeared to be a deadly threat, the USDA did put in a legal action to seize the product—but only at *one* location where the damage was discovered. Meanwhile, dealers' shelves throughout the country were stacked up and waiting for the unprotected consumer.

One case in 1963 concerned a rodent-control formula containing thallium sulphate, a paste that looks like peanut butter. Tragedy whipped across the country to fell 400 persons, many of whom died and most of whom were children. USDA finally got around to canceling registration of the product two years later, in 1965. But it failed to withdraw any of the product that was already on the market. The USDA never even bothered to find out where the thallium products were registered, even though there were forty-five companies making the substance and over fifty-eight different kinds on the market across the country.

The story of USDA involving Shell Oil's No-Pest Strip, those tidy-looking, orange-colored cardboard boxes that are so innocently hung in millions of homes and restaurants to keep flies away, is a strong candidate for the raised-eyebrow department.

Vapona, the base of the No-Pest Strip, and lindane, the component of the electrical-type pesticide dispenser, silently dispel a continuous amount of invisible pesticide into the atmosphere of whatever room they are in, permeating and covering everything and anybody in the room with an unnoticeable residue. In the summer of 1966, the Public Health Service objected strenuously to Shell's No-Pest Strip, stating that "We do not recommend the registration of this registered number because the devices used, deliberately subject human beings to continued exposure to a pesticide. Furthermore, the type of device is non-discriminatory, in that it subjects both humans and insects to the same concentration of the pesticides."

USDA's Agricultural Research Service registered the product anyway, and the Public Health Service watered down its demands, provided that the Shell Oil Company would include a warning for the consumer not to use the product in rooms occupied by infants or infirm individuals. The same phrase had been used for the electric dispenser that wafted out the fumes of lindane.

The USDA section handling this sort of thing was headed up by Dr. Harry W. Hays, who confessed that he didn't see the need to bother recalling all the Shell vapona strips on shelves all over the country to put this warning on the product, even though Shell's No-Pest Strip registration required that the warning be there in plain view. What's more, Dr. Hays took no action whatever to make it known to the public that the Shell strips could be hazardous. When it came to animals, the USDA was most solicitous in its warnings. For example, the USDA had taken great pains to publicize a Pfizer vaccine that had been hazardous to cattle. For the Shell strip, the agency apparently didn't think a warning was necessary.

Interesting in the case is that another vapona product very similar to Shell's No-Pest produced by the Aeroseal Company had much rougher going at the hands of the USDA. On the surface, the reasons were rather unclear. For some period of time, Aeroseal bought its vapona from Shell but later decided to manufacture its own product altogether. Even though the basic ingredient was the same as Shell's No-Pest, the USDA decided to cancel its privileges and yanked the Aeroseal product off the market, while Shell's remained on. The yanking process took exactly four days, something of a record for the USDA. Similar cases averaged around fifteen months. Most interesting is that the recall could be traced directly to a complaint by Shell.

Noteworthy also was that, although it took only four days to get Aeroseal off the market entirely, it took some eight letters from the Public Health Service to the USDA to get Shell to agree to put the simple and vitally necessary warning statement on No-Pest. Meantime, mothers would be content to put the Shell strips over a baby's crib and feel that the infant was safe and sound.

The Shell No-Pest Strip fills the room with vapor. Since restaurant and other foods automatically are covered with an invisible residue, it raises the legal question that anyone producing such a device should have it cleared with the FDA for establishing an acceptable residue level. The product, in other words, creates residues on foods served by restaurants to the public and becomes an uninvited food additive. The USDA had not filed any request to the FDA for such a tolerance, but since the law itself is vague on the point, the situation is somewhat confused. The fact remains that the strip contaminates any food exposed to it, to say nothing of people. It is also strange that the USDA permits Shell No-Pest Strips to be used freely in the home, nursery, and restaurant —but prohibits its use in meat packing and processing plants. Which should get higher priority of protection? Babies or meat?

Underneath the surface of the story that found Shell sitting in such a privileged position, issuing from the largess of the USDA, is the appointment by Dr. Hays of Dr. T. Roy Hansberry to a special task force to study USDA procedures on registering pesticides. It so happened that Dr. Hansberry was an official of a Shell Chemical Company research affiliate. Personnel records at the USDA indicated that Dr. Hansberry had no official business with any firm which might constitute a conflict of interest—although, of course, Shell is one of the largest producers of pesticides in the country.

Dr. Hansberry found himself, of all things, sitting on a special three-man committee which reviewed the manner in which pesticide registration applications should be approved.

Another consultant on the USDA rolls from 1963 to 1969 was Dr. Mitchell Zavon. At the same time he was carrying out these responsibilities, he was also serving as a medical consultant to the Shell Chemical Company. Oddly enough, Dr. Zavon conducted a number of scientific studies on vapona, and Shell used them to support its claims that the Shell No-Pest Strips were totally safe. The foods that Dr. Zavon submitted to the Shell labs after exposure to the strips were pure and faultless, with not a sign of any vapona residues. Strangely, studies by outside scientists showed that the strips unquestionably left residues on food exposed to them.

All through the conflict, Shell was complaining. It formally objected to the Public Health Service studies. At first, Shell tried to rewrite the label warning to make it sound soft and innocuous. When the Public Health Service refused to go along with this, Shell petulantly insisted again that no warning was needed, asserting that they had new data and that USDA's Dr. Hays "didn't see the need" for revising the label.

But by January, 1969, even the USDA was getting stubborn, under pressure from the Public Health Service. They insisted that Shell comply with a label that read: "Do not use in nurseries or rooms where infants, ill or aged persons are confined." But Shell kept fighting. They wanted to use the words "continuously confined"—which, of course, subtly suggested that the strip could still be used safely over a baby's crib or an invalid's bed. This, however, was unacceptable, and finally Shell gave in on January 8, 1969, stating that it didn't agree but that it would comply.

But one important thing was still omitted: The label contained no warning about the contamination of food. Finally, the legend was added: "Do not use in kitchens, restaurants, or areas where food is prepared and served"—this legend being forced by the FDA's review of the problem and the hazards involved.

There are some postscripts to the story. It was recommended by a Congressional committee that the cases of Dr. Hansberry, Dr. Zavon, and a former USDA pharmacologist named John Leary concerning conflict of interest be referred to the Department of Justice.

The discovery of vapona (DDVP is another name for it) was made in a laboratory of the Public Health Service's Communicable Disease Center. Under careful control, and with proper warning about its use, it is a powerful and effective insecticide. Since it had been discovered by government scientists, an article in *Public Health Reports* dedicated the free use of the product to any manufacturer.

Shell Chemical Company felt differently. It decided to claim exclusive U.S. patent rights.

Residues of DDT have been found in penguins in Antarctica, with the nearest use of the product thousands of miles away. A coho salmon catch from Lake Michigan—15,000 pounds of it—was riddled with prohibitive DDT levels. Mice fed a heavy diet of DDT became cancerous. Recent studies show that 25 percent of all DDT made has now ended up in the seas. Endrin, used to protect cotton and other crops, killed thousands of fish in the lower Mississippi. These and other persistent "hard" pesticides have created a problem that will last for generations, even though DDT's use is considerably squelched as of this moment. Nearly everyone knows the story, but even the experts don't really know what to do about it.

Hope for an escape from the iron grasp on the environment by DDT was stimulated when "softer" pesticides were developed, pesticides that break down quicker after use, are not cumulative, and eventually fade away.

There was great hope when Parathion came along, because it was so "soft." But accidental poisonings from Parathion have been so lethal and so persistent that enthusiasm for it has died along with the victims. Parathion is a triple-threat product. It can kill when consumed, inhaled, or spilled on the skin. Even the USDA is a little startled about it, going to elaborate lengths in designing new labels, tags, and posters to warn about its dangers. But the agency still resists banning it.

One of the unhealthiest controversies in recent times is the one that centers around the herbicide 2,4,5-T. If a search were on to find great industrial statesmanship, it would be better not to include the Hercules Corporation or Dow Chemical on the list. As two manufacturers of this herbicide, they have been enjoying an enormous volume of sales to the Pentagon for use in literally decimating the Vietnam landscape, subjecting thousands of civilians to possible birth defects, and fighting off even the feeble attempts of the USDA and FDA to put some kind of clamp on the domestic sales of this poison. As far as the concern of these companies regarding biological warfare, it has never been expressed.

It took a group of young law students from Nader's Raiders to bring the lurking dangers of 2,4,5-T to the surface, after they had discovered a report from Bionetics, a laboratory working on contract for the National Cancer Institute, buried in the FDA files. It had been lying around for months, since February, 1969. It was midsummer when the report was found. The report revealed that 2,4,5-T produced birth defects in mice, a serious harbinger of trouble. Even though the report was channeled to the USDA, the FDA, and the Department of Defense, no action was taken by these agencies to warn the public of the potential danger. Meanwhile, the use of the chemical continued to increase in food growing, residential lawn control, and other everyday uses throughout the country as a brush and weed killer of tremendous potency. It wasn't until the end of October, 1969, that Dr. Lee A. DuBridge, director of the White House Office of Science and Technology, publicly announced that the USDA would cancel all registration on the chemical for use on food crops. (He did nothing to restrict its use around homes and gardens.)

DuBridge's statement was a masterpiece of double talk. Thomas Whiteside, who was responsible for propelling a lot of Congressional action through Senator Hart's subcommittee dealing with environmental problems, wrote in an article in *The New Yorker*:

> In certain respects, the DuBridge announcement is a curious document. In its approach to the facts about 2,4,5-T that were set forth in the Bionetics report, it reflects considerable sensitivity to the political and international issues that lie behind the widespread use of this powerful herbicide for civilian and military purposes, and the words in which it describes the reason for restricting its use appear to have been very carefully chosen.

DuBridge referred to "relatively large oral doses" given to the laboratory animals. As Whiteside documented, this was somewhat of an understatement. According to an eminent biologist, the dosages of 21.5 and 46.4 milligrams per kilogram of the body weights fed to the rats studied and the percentage of abnormal fetuses being 90 to 100 percent would hardly justify DuBridge's statement above or his further statement that these were merely a "higher than expected number of deformities." It was a *massive* number of deformities.

Nor did the President's science adviser see fit to mention the malformed animals born after a 2,4,5-T spraying by the U.S. Forest Service in the Tonto National Forest in Arizona, to say nothing of the people in the area who came down with symptoms associated with herbicide poisoning. The regional forestry commissioner who conducted the spraying operation said he knew nothing about the problems with 2,4,5-T until he read it in the papers.

Harrison Wellford, of Ralph Nader's group, conducted a survey to see if the ban against 2,4,5-T was effective against its sale in the Washington, D.C., area. His team covered fifteen retail stores. One-third of them were still selling the prohibited products, even though the USDA had requested a recall. The products included Real-Kill Spot Weed Killer, Amchem Weed-on, Greenfield Crab Grass Broadleaf Weed Killer, Ortho Weed-be-gon Spot Weeder, and Ortho Brush Killer—all in liquid form and forbidden around the home, on water, or in recreation areas.

The USDA also got around to canceling the use of the dry form of 2,4,5-T, but Hercules and Dow Chemical, joined by Amchem, appealed the ban. They can continue to produce and sell this poison pending the outcome. Hercules even went further. It protested the ban on liquid 2,4,5-T.

One of the most dangerous loopholes left open by the ban is that Silvex, an extremely popular herbicide for backyard use, was not banned, along with others that are of the same chemical family. Silvex involves the same ingredient that was found to produce serious birth defects in 2,4,5-T, known as dioxin—not that pure 2,4,5-T does not produce the defects alone. Without Silvex being banned, the public can easily be deceived that this product is a safe substitute for 2,4,5-T.

The same USDA story began emerging as in the Shell No-Pest situation. By permitting the dry form of 2,4,5-T to remain on the market, the ban had little real effect. By permitting Silvex to remain, the public was lulled into a feeling of false safety. By not publishing the ban in the *Federal Register*, the ban was ineffective. By sending out a form letter to manufacturers of the chemical, the USDA left a loophole whereby some of the products could remain on the market by relabeling to eliminate some of the "claims." By not making public a specific list of trade names involved, the USDA

made it impossible for the consumer to know which herbicides are safe and which are not.

Harrison Wellford and several other individuals and
groups joined to petition the USDA to correct these and
other deficiencies. Among the petitioners was Mrs. Lorraine
Huber, of Bethesda, Maryland, who is a registered nurse.
Her three-year-old daughter was playing in the yard one
day, when a large dosage of 2,4,5-T drifted over from another yard. The child went through a long, drawn-out period
of physical and mental illness as a result of inhaling the
fumes of the chemical. One more exposure to the chemical
could be fatal for the child.

Cited in the petition is the appearance of gross malforma-
tions in human babies after the U.S. Air Force's intense soaking of the Vietnam countryside by *50,000 tons* of herbicides.

There are other stories, equally harrowing. Dow Chemical
had to shut down its 2,4,5-T plant in Midland, Michigan,
after sixty workers came down with chloracne, a persistent
disease for which there is no known treatment and which
causes large skin eruptions, liver damage, disorders of the
central nervous system, chronic fatigue, and depression.
Three Vietnamese citizens died when sprayed with 2,4,5-T.
Spray from aerial treatment of crops has been known to drift
as far as 100 miles. One dust storm carried 2,4,5-T all the
way from southern Texas to Cincinnati, Ohio. Even without
a wind, children playing in a yard are likely to be exposed
from as far as 100 yards away. The chemical can take as long
as a year to break down and disappear. There is actually *no*
safe method for use.

But this did not seem to bother the Hercules Corporation.
In early February, 1971, it announced with great fanfare
that a series of tests that the company had contracted with
the Bionetics Laboratories showed clearly that its tests directly contradicted the findings of the National Institute of
Environmental Health Sciences. These were the tests that
had led to the eventual USDA ban on 2,4,5-T and that had
blasted the controversy wide open.

The government tests had shown that the chemical was unquestionably the cause of severe birth defects in laboratory animals. How could the new tests conducted for Hercules oppose these carefully-arrived-at conclusions?

Hercules immediately asked the new Environmental Protection Agency, which had just now assumed responsibility for this sort of pesticide function, to stop action immediately on suspending the use of 2,4,5-T.

Hercules officials contacting EPA Administrator William D. Ruckelshaus heartily claimed that there were no birth defects whatever in ten litters of a laboratory strain known as Charles River laboratory mice. The same samples were tested in a different solution, and still, the Hercules officials claimed, there were no birth defects in eleven litters of the mice.

The National Institute of Environmental Health tests had shown strikingly different results. Nine pregnant mice had come up with a 32.9-percent incidence of cleft palate and a 12.3-percent incidence of severe kidney disorders in the fetuses.

Hercules concluded its statement by saying that the new experiments "all failed to confirm teratogenicity [birth defects, from the Greek word meaning "monster"] even at the excessive doses of 100 milligrams per kilogram daily subcutaneously administered."

This was serious stuff. If Hercules was right, the removal of the product would be a gross mistake. Millions of lives and dollars were at stake.

It took about three weeks to straighten out the mystery. The sample doses used in the Hercules tests were—"by error," we are told—*exactly ten times weaker* than the 100 milligrams per kilogram used in the government tests, a standard supported by nearly all the scientists involved in the issue.

With its tail between its legs, Hercules admitted it was all just a big mistake. But it still didn't give up. Along with Dow Chemical and Shell and others, it was opposing any new legislation that would give the new Environmental Protection Agency any new powers to protect the consumer. "We believe," said J. G. Copeland, general manager of Hercules' Synthetics Department, "that Congress should not give a new agency any more power until the need for such broad powers is first demonstrated."

If the need for broad regulatory powers has not been demonstrated by now in the actions of the pesticide manufacturers, it never will be. However, the USDA seemed more interested in the loss farmers might face if 2,4,5-T were completely banned: about $52,000,000, or approximately the cost of one destroyer. The USDA made no mention of the possibility of babies with twisted bodies, of children stricken on backyard lawns, or of workers covered with grotesque, untreatable acne. Nor did they mention what FDA's Dr. Jacqueline Verrett told a Congressional committee about one of 2,4,5-T's most potent components, tetradioxin. Speaking of the comparison of the effect on chicks and mammals between this and thalidomide, she said: "You would have to say this material is 100,000 to a million times more potent in these particular species."

What has never been mentioned in all the confusion and controversy about 2,4,5-T is the close relationship between this herbicide and the chemical hexachlorophene, which has been permeating personal use items like Dial soap, pHiso-Hex, Johnson & Johnson First Aid Cream, feminine sprays, cosmetics, toothpastes, mouthwashes, and dozens of other products used daily by almost the entire population.

The new and later developments on that story bear close scrutiny and will be found in the pages that follow.

13

Home Sweet Home?

EVERY house is an island surrounded by floating hazards. Many of them are so common, they are hardly thought of or noticed until sudden injury or death strikes the family. Protection from household hazards is as scanty and thin and irregular as it is with the loopholes and blindspots in the food, drug, and cosmetic areas, if not more so.

The full story of what happened with the "innocent" household dry cleaner carbon tetrachloride illustrates through stark tragedy how lack of government action can drag out when major hazards are staring the protection agencies in the face for years. This kind of story can be happening now—in several areas.

The innocuous-sounding label appearing on carbon tet containers meant practically nothing to the consumer. There was no explanation of what "adequate ventilation" really was. What should have been on the label during the nearly seventy years this product was a byword around the house (as in foods, a GRAS item if there ever was one) was a statement: *"The chances are this product will kill you."*

It took from 1902 to the 1930's for the medical profession to begin to feel that maybe it wasn't too good an idea to use carbon tet in medical practice, as it had been doing up until the beginning of the century. It had been used as an anesthetic, in spite of the report one doctor wrote: "The boundary between insensibility and death appears to be so narrow and ill-defined as in practice not to be capable of regulation." In spite of this, doctors recommended it orally as a good way to get rid of hookworm. Enthusiastic articles in the medical journals of the day supported this idea. By the 1930's, however, the series of deaths and injuries that followed this practice began to provide a few hints that all was not well with this inspired idea. Perhaps the medical journal editors had not run across some of the data that had accumulated in the early 1900's, when women found carbon tet as the ideal agent for dry shampoos. The hair and scalp were enjoying an excellent dry-cleaning process, but women by the dozens were toppling from the fumes, many of them never to live again. The women had the sense to give it up by the time 1913 rolled around.

But industry and home use went merrily along. As a metal degreaser, a solvent for rubber cement, a fumigant for grain, a replacement of naphtha for dry cleaning and for the manufacture of soaps, printing inks, and freon gases for refrigerants, carbon tet enjoyed a splendid and unsullied reputation. Even a long series of poisonings and deaths in the rubber cement factories failed to dim the enthusiasm of its supporters. The deaths came, it was thought, simply because of inadequate ventilation.

By 1933, there were some 10,000,000 carbon tet fire extinguishers in use, many of them the type that look like large light bulbs hanging on wall brackets. When the temperature reaches a certain level, the glass bulb crashes to the floor and is supposed to put out the fire underneath it. What the extinguisher manufacturers failed to emphasize was that the vapor rising from flames and carbon tet were about as deadly as you could assemble in one place.

Even the two welders in 1919 who were unwilling guinea pigs failed to precipitate corrective action. Working in a compartment of a Navy submarine in Portsmouth, one of the workers found his clothing ignited by a slice of hot metal. His fellow worker grabbed a carbon tet fire extinguisher and sprayed him with it. The fire was extinguished immediately, but both men dropped to the floor unconscious from the fumes. Rescue workers had to cut their way into the compartment, then rushed the men to the hospital. One died within five days, the other in nine. The cause of the deaths was recorded as poisoning from carbon tet vapors.

The tragedy was punctuated by the monstrous facts that emerged later. It was discovered that when carbon tet is exposed to high temperature, it obliges by forming the deadly phosgene gas, which was used in World War I as one of its most lethal weapons.

This tragedy happened in 1919. It would be thought that with the discovery of the phosgene gas by-product every such fire extinguisher would have been seized and destroyed in both homes and factories. Instead, production increased and sales proliferated. *It took until July, 1967,* for the Underwriters Laboratories to withdraw its listing of carbon tet extinguishers as qualifying for use of their U.L. label. In 1970, the product was *still* in use.

Since 1962, only one company has had the gall to produce this type of extinguisher, the General Fire Extinguishing Company. Aiding and abetting this lethal imposition on the user was the Dow Chemical Company from its Freeport, Texas, plant. Jointly, both companies stated that they "discouraged" distributors from selling the carbon tetrachloride extinguishers and refills to noncommercial customers, but there was no positive control over the product beyond the branch office level.

If carbon tet was an insidious killer as a fire extinguisher, it was far more deadly and pervasive as a household cleaner. For years, the consumer felt that it was a relatively safe cleaner, and the mild warnings on the label suggesting adequate ventilation were honored more in the breach than in the practice. The danger was increased by the fact that inhalation of the fumes was much more apt to cause death and injury than by swallowing or skin exposure.

All through the long years since 1902 it has been freely available at drug and hardware stores, with little hint of its general dangers and no hint of its exaggerated effect on obese persons or those who have been having a few drinks before using it. The problem with the "adequate ventilation" warning is this: Simply opening doors and windows will not do. The only way for real protection would be to install an expensive and commercial-type exhaust vent system that no householder has at his fingertips. By the late 1940's, well-ventilated industrial plants gave up the use of the fluid because of multiple injuries and deaths. Even the giant industrial exhaust systems could not cope with the problem. Further, by the time a user is aware of the seductive odor of carbon tet, it has already reached a concentration of 80 parts per million—exactly eight times greater than the tolerance level. In other words, the consumer would be already hit by deadly levels before he got any hint of the odor. One teaspoon of carbon tet in a small bathroom will produce a concentration vapor of 100 parts per million. A half a pint dropped on the floor would produce over 4,000—a fatal gulp of the fumes.

It doesn't take much doing. In May, 1968, a man did a quick cleaning job on his necktie in his kitchen. He threw up that evening, came down with chills and fever the next day, and over the next three days he became increasingly nervous, worked up, and restless. His breathing rate increased markedly, and he went to a Boston hospital on May 16. By the next day, he was dead from acute hepatic necrosis and renal failure due to inhaling carbon tet. The doctors and the hospital were useless: There is *no* treatment or antidote whatever for the poisoning.

Even more tragic was the case involving the seven-year-old son of a California chemical engineer. His wife, rising later than usual on a Sunday morning, went into the child's bedroom to find him and his four-year-old brother unconscious on the floor. She quickly called her husband, who immediately detected carbon tet fumes. The four-year-old was revived by a rescue squad; the seven-year-old was dead on arrival at the hospital. The area of the rug where the boys were found lying was soaked, and a towel smelling of carbon tet lay nearby. They had apparently been trying to clean something that had spilled on the rug in their room.

If the carbon tet story points up the time bomb situation in common household products, the story of the Relaxacisor does an equally impressive job in chilling the enthusiasm for health and reducing gadgets that are spawned in the market with little thought on the part of the manufacturer. Unlike drugs or food additives, household substances, toys, cosmetics, and many other hazards need no clearance whatever from any agency before they are scattered across the country on the market. The only recourse the FDA has is to prove a legal case or to seize one shipment at a time, at great expense and with infinite delays.

If you were one of the 400,000 persons who bought a Relaxacisor, you would not be cheered by the growing number of users who began to develop or aggravate many serious physical conditions from the use of the machine. The Relaxacisor came in battery or plug-in models and supplied electrical shocks that produced forty muscle contractions a minute through contact pads that were placed on various parts of the body. Ostensibly, this was supposed to exercise these parts and to reduce the waistline. The Relaxacisor manufacturer managed to build into the machine factors that were extremely hazardous and definitely contraindicated in conditions such as intraabdominal, gastrointestinal, orthopedic, muscular, neurological, vascular, kidney, gynecological, and pelvic disorders. Cancer cells that were dormant could be activated and spread by the electrical gyrations produced by the machine through its violent and unnatural movements. People with epilepsy, hernia, multiple sclerosis, ulcers, and other conditions could be irreversibly damaged.

The machines cost anywhere from $100 to $400 and were matched by similar ones made by other companies. All of them worked on the principle that made the body part of an electrical circuit. When an FDA warning went out, it applied to all machines of this type except those used under direct medical supervision.

The tragic part about the case is that it took nearly a decade for the FDA to get the device off the market, and then only after a five-month trial involving forty victims and many prominent medical experts. If the same laws were in effect for medical devices as for drugs, the machine would never have reached the market because the burden of proof for safety and effectiveness would have been on the manufacturer. A sad postscript to the story is that many of those who had bought the machine attempted to unload the product secondhand through classified ads.

Warnings also went out on an electronic neuromuscular stimulater called the Batronic Ventilaide, which was supposed to be an artificial respiration device. While the manufacturer, the Batrow Laboratories of Branford, Connecticut, finally agreed to stop further distribution, the company refused to recall those devices already on the market. In late 1970, the FDA began the painfully slow process of seizure action.

On one July morning not too long ago, an eighteen-month-old boy by the name of Mike Snodgrass was toddling about the kitchen of his home. It was seven thirty in the morning. His father had left for work, his mother was in a nearby room, and his older brother, Wayne, was in the next room. Suddenly, Wayne heard young Mike choking and gagging. He rushed in and called his mother, who joined him in seconds. The door under the kitchen sink next to the electric dishwasher was wide open. Beside Mike was a box of Finish detergent, made for electrical dishwashing. The spout of the box was open, and Mike's mouth was full of the powder. His mother, who had once studied nursing, grabbed the boy, put him over the kitchen sink, and rinsed his mouth out.

Then she called the Poison Control Center. They were not too well up on detergents but felt Mrs. Snodgrass had done the right thing. However, they did advise her to take the child to his doctor.

At the pediatrician's office, the doctor studied Mike's throat closely. He advised that Mike be kept home under close observation but did not send him to the hospital.

By noon, he had a fever. His mouth and lips were blistered. Mike was brought back to the doctor for X rays. But even before the X rays could be developed, Mike's condition became rapidly worse. Without delay, he was rushed to a children's hospital about eight miles away. On the way, his breathing became more and more labored. He was rushed directly to the emergency room and remained in surgery for over six hours.

Here a tube was put into his throat for breathing and one into his stomach. Several times, it looked as if he were going to expire.

The prognosis was several months in the hospital and probably major surgery on the esophagus. Young Mike had to have restraints on his arms, because he would constantly try to pull the tubes out of his mouth and stomach. Each time this happened, a panic situation came up.

But several months later, he miraculously began to recuperate. It was hard to believe, and the doctors were incredulous. Mike was brought home in October. For several weeks, things seemed to be going well. Then he began having trouble in swallowing and breathing. Soon he could hardly swallow at all. He was rushed to the hospital for surgery.

Open-neck surgery of this sort usually requires a skin graft on the throat, using membrane taken from the patient's own intestines. But a last-minute idea of the surgeon's avoided this through probing under the lip of the scar tissue. Mike's esophagus had been twisted to one side by the scar tissue healing over the opening.

With his trach and gastrostomy tubes, Mike was able to be brought home by Christmas. A vaporizer was kept going constantly in his room. Night after night, his parents would listen for sounds of trouble. His mother would have to apply a suction device to Mike's trach tube every few hours, night and day. Several times, he would pull out the tubes, and he would have to be rushed to the hospital to have them reinserted. In March, nine months after the accident, he came down with severe bronchial congestion and had to be brought back to the hospital for another stay. After he was released, more trouble developed on the anniversary of the accident. Each week he would have to return to have small notches cut into the edge of the scar tissue in his throat. The future is hopeful but still uncertain.

This story is far from an isolated case. Small children are sitting ducks for any of the fifty different chemicals sitting around the average household. Drugs and medicines account for about half of the poisonings of the toddlers, with aspirin being the most frequent villain. Cleaning and polishing agents are next in line, especially furniture polish. Children aspirate these petroleum distillates into the lungs as they drink the fluid. Chemical pneumonitis can set in in a matter of minutes, and deaths are not infrequent. Often the polish has an attractive fragrance and an enticing color and thus becomes what is legally termed an "attractive nuisance."

Many children who eat lye are not as lucky as Mike. A lot of them die from shock, infection, or perforation of the esophagus or stomach. Dr. Glen E. Wegner, of HEW, tells of a household drain cleaner that is made up of 94-percent concentrated sulfuric acid. It is packed in a tightly-capped plastic container. Two people have tried to force the cap open, and in doing so the liquid splashed open with great force, covering the face, eyes, and neck and causing severe burns.

Other products, seemingly innocuous to the adult, can be deadly with children: cosmetics, turpentine, paints, pesticides, petroleum products, and even flowering plants. (In the Southeast, kerosene kept in a Coke bottle is often a poisoning cause.) Almost one child dies every day from household poisoning in this country.

The worst ages for a child are from one to four years. He's able to move about quickly, has really no critical judgment, and he likes to put everything he can get his hands on into his mouth. In the face of protests from anxious mothers throughout the country, who are most verbal, Congress has been trying to create legislation that will call for child-proof packaging of dangerous products—all, of course, in the face of the usual unerringly predictable industry opposition.

Of interest is the child known as the "Pica" child, which is Latin for "magpie." He is prone to eat any nonfood substance he can find. According to Dr. Roger Meyer, of the Northwestern University Medical School, this type of child has to be carefully watched. Once he is poisoned and recovers, he has a four times greater chance of repeating the process. He uses it as a device for gaining attention and for the excitement of another trip to the hospital.

Dr. Meyer also points out that poisoning incidents don't occur around the clock at random times. Most of them take place between 3 and 6 P.M., when the child is hungry and the mothers are busy. Early morning is also a critical time.

Television commercials about pills and drugs don't help at all. They condition the child to think that it's just the thing to do, and quite a social occasion at times. Dr. Meyer tells of a five-year-old who lined up a long row of aspirin tablets and started his baby brother off on a race from the other end to see who could eat the most pills.

In the face of all this, you would think that industry would be in favor of the bill that Senator Frank E. Moss and co-sponsor Senator Warren G. Magnuson were sponsoring, known as the Poison Prevention Packaging Act of 1969. In its simplest terms, it was shaped to give the Secretary of Health, Education, and Welfare power to set standards for packaging designed to prevent young children from getting at hazardous substances found around the house.

Not that labeling means anything to the very young child, and warnings on dangerous products are generally tucked away on the label in about the most inaccessible place you can find. But Leon Wolfstone, president of the American Trial Lawyers Association, noted that often a product like a dry-cleaning fluid has a label worded in a quiet and overgentlemanly way, suggesting that it's better to use the product in a well-ventilated room. The blunt, direct "killer" label is often obligatory but always protested against by the manufacturer.

Young children can't read, but they can have certain pictures impressed on their brains, especially if they have shock value. Attorney Wolfstone would go so far as to recommend that a picture of a coffin with a child in it would not be too much of an overstatement on the label for such serious matters.

Threatened with the possibility of vigorous legislation, the chemical, patent medicines, and similar establishment companies retorted with some of the strangest logic that has yet been concocted. Dr. Maurice Tainter, a vice-president of Sterling Drug, makers of Bayer Aspirin, indicated that even though aspirin is involved in more accidental poisoning episodes than any other individual drug or group of products, ". . . the remedy proposed in the pending legislation is not timely, nor likely to be really effective, nor to promote public welfare."

He went on to say: "We [the manufacturers] are confident that if we are not restrained or inhibited by well-intended but premature legislation, we will continue to make conspicuous gains in the years ahead . . . this is not the time for new legislation or regulation which well might have the adverse effect of checking the valuable progress now being made."

The Bayer representative failed to explain why little or nothing had been done before or especially in the early sixties, for instance, when deaths from aspirin or aspirin compounds were soaring to the highest peak in history. He tried to explain to Senator Moss how child safety standards set by the HEW would retard "the valuable progress now being made," but his reasoning was very hard to follow.

"This is a matter of practical human experience," the Bayer Aspirin man explained. "If you [HEW and Congress] establish standards which say that a safety closure [safety cap for a bottle] has to meet a certain performance standard, and we succeed in producing such a safety closure, we will use that closure to fulfill the law and the requirements. Then our attempts to develop better closures will probably stop or be minimal from there on."

Just why such apathy would set in at Sterling Drug Company in its Bayer Aspirin operations he failed to explain satisfactorily. His argument, in effect, would indicate that the minimum standards for auto tires would prevent tire companies from going ahead to make better tires. Or the requirements for seat belts in autos would stop auto manufacturers from making other improvements. The more he tried to explain his opposition, the more confused he got, with such statements as: "If you get the Government in there telling you you have to do it at this level as a minimum, it takes away a lot of the competitive urge."

Senator Moss responded: ". . . you say to me, well, if the Government comes along and sets a standard . . . we will take it and we will just forget about whether children are dying, whether they are being poisoned. We will just abandon all that."

Dr. Tainter's ineloquent plea for Bayer Aspirin was no less confused than the arguments against the new safety packaging protection bill by the Proprietary Association, representing the leading manufacturers of patent medicines, a phrase that turns the members livid when they hear it. "We think," said the association's spokesman, "the legislative requirements contemplated by this bill would better come at a later time when studies and experimentation now in progress have advanced further." He did not explain why self-regulation had not advanced further all through the years when children like Mike Snodgrass were getting into deadly household substances constantly—and continue to do so. He did not explain the way this new delay would prevent the continuation of the child-poisoning incidents.

The patent medicine men were joined in outlook and attitude by the Chemical Specialties Manufacturers Association, which stated that "It is keenly mindful that this delegation of exceedingly broad authority may create very serious problems for the industry with only speculative and doubtful benefits for the public." The Pharmaceutical Manufacturers Association, back at the same old stand, said: "We have serious doubts that enactment of such legislation at the present time would be in the public interest."

Most of the 285,013 cases of accidental swallowing of household products by children under five between 1966 and 1969 occurred because the toddlers were able to open containers, according to the FDA. Why did industry fight laws to prevent this?

Fortunately, all the piety and wit of the various industrial associations failed in their attempts to block the act. It became the Poison Prevention Packaging Act of 1970, its final approval by Congress barely squeezing into that calendar year, on December 30.

The Reverend John R. Dryer, pastor of the Covenant Church of Wellsville, Ohio, was proud of his baby son and made sure that he would have the best possible care. He was particularly impressed with the Kiddie Koop playpen-crib. Its manufacturers proudly published the slogan: "Since 1912. Your baby's health, safety, and comfort are our only business."

Reverend Dryer decided to buy the Kiddie Koop because its netted lining would keep out mosquitoes and other bugs. In contrast, the cheaper cribs and playpens had slots which seemed to leave room for a baby's head to poke through. What's more, the Kiddie Koop had a lid that would stop his one-year-old from tumbling out and, of course, complete the protection from the bugs. The lid was held by a long metal hinge in addition to plastic straps that encircled the lid.

One morning, Reverend Dryer came into his baby's nursery and found the lid partway open. In the space between the lid and the side of the crib was the baby's head. The baby was dead, strangled.

Because of the warm weather, the plastic straps had stretched, making it possible for the baby to push his head up into the crack between the lid and the crib side. The more the infant tried to pull away, the more firmly the lid clamped his neck, and the tighter the side clamped on his throat.

The devastated father pleaded with the manufacturer either to make the Kiddie Koop safe or to take it off the market. All the company would do was to extend its "sympathy."

Just three and a half weeks before this tragedy happened, a nine-month-old son of a policeman in Coral Gables, Florida, was strangled in the same kind of crib and under the same circumstances. The Kiddie Koop continued to remain on the market.

Crib strangulation accounts for up to 4 deaths per 100 of the recorded deaths in Boston. In Los Angeles, 15 to 20 out of 250 deaths each year are caused by "mechanical compression of infants"—or crib strangulation.

Accidental deaths among children under fifteen years of age come to 15,000. This is higher than the deaths from cancer, contagious diseases, heart diseases, and gastroenteritis combined.

Many parents have the notion that some big government agency in the sky is seeing to it that no hazardous toys or baby furniture and the like are put on the market. This is far from true, even though the Toy Safety Act of 1969 has now been put into effect. Again, the act affords none of the protection that drugs and food additive laws provide. There is no preclearance—only long, laborious legal action such as that in the infinitely long, drawn-out case of the Relaxacisor. Meanwhile, the toy maker can continue blissfully to flood the market with anything that sells well.

The National Commission on Product Safety has collected just a few samples of the letters it receives from the public regarding toys on the market that eventually bring dubious joy to the child who gets them:

Item: Ideal toy balloon. "A balloon was broken with such force that a fragment shot her eye, and vision was blurred for two days."

Item: Cradle Symphony Musical Toy. "Apparently while taking a rest in bed, the loop went around the baby's neck and hooked on to the bar and the baby's struggling only made the loop tighter and he was found dead in bed with obvious signs of strangulation."

Item: Thayer Play Pen. "When my baby was four months old he rolled over from his stomach to his back and wedged his head in the V-support of the play pen. Luckily, I was in the next room and responded to his cries immediately."

Item: Little Lady Oven. "Temperatures on the sides of this oven reach 200° F, on the top 300° and higher, and the inside shelf heated to 660°, a temperature in excess of that reached by the ordinary household oven."

Item: Metal casting set. "Temperatures reached 800° on the inside of the stove which is accessible when the ladle is not in place, and 500° to 600° on surfaces that could be touched even with the ladle in place. Clothing and other combustible material could easily catch fire in such circumstances. Moreover, the set developed a potentially lethal shock hazard during testing."

Item: Zulu Dart Blow Guns. "Eleven children in Philadelphia had to have small one-inch plastic darts with sharpened needles in them removed from their lungs when they inhaled them instead of blowing them out of this dart gun."

The carnage is not confined to home and household toys. Stationary recreational equipment brings more than squeals of delight with it. Yearly injury estimates run 500,000 injuries from swings, 200,000 from slides, 50,000 from seesaws.

Other items that are on the market are by no means a mother's joy. Chemical sets have been found with inadequate or nonexistent caution labels. The deadly poisonous jequirity beans have not only been sold in necklaces but in other jewelry, rosaries, and dolls' eyes. One bead chewed and swallowed could be fatal.

Much tragedy could be avoided if distributors and retailers anticipated dangers in children's merchandise and refused to offer them for sale. In Baltimore, a two-year-old infant was presented with a pacifier made in Hong Kong, smaller than American models, and which had a ramrod effect when pushed into the mouth. The child died from strangulation. A good many collapsible, spring-supported infant seats, known as walker-jumpers or baby bouncers and nationally distributed, have amputated babies' fingers and lacerated hands and faces. Nearly 500,000 of these are sold every year. Nine baby finger amputations have resulted from the baby putting his finger into the springs or X-shaped pivot areas of the frame. Unguarded springs and lack of a safety

iock are another hazard. Tilting or tipping can also cause
dangerous accidents.

The importer who brought in "cracker balls," or ball-type
caps, deserves a medal of limited distinction. These look exactly like candy balls, or even the dry cereals of this sort, and
they explode on impact. They were often sold at candy coun-
ters. Over thirty children, at least, bit on them, to shatter and
burn gums, tongue, and inner cheek, to say nothing of loos-
ening teeth. Before the Toy Safety Act, the FDA could not
ban imports.

The toy business is big business. Its sales range between
$2.5 and $3 billion a year—about thirty times the entire
FDA budget in recent years.

When Senator Moss' consumer subcommittee began pushing through the Toy Safety Act in 1969, the usual happened.
This time it was the Toy Manufacturers of America. The organization is dominated by the big ones: Hasbro Industries,
Remco, Ideal, Mattel, Milton Bradley, and many others. In
trying to block the Safety Act, the association's official statement said: "The precipitate speed with which this proposed
legislation has been drafted and brought to hearing should
not be allowed to create the impression that we face an emergency or a crisis in the matter of toy safety. . . . There is no
evidence of any emergency."

Then Jerome Fryer, speaking for the Toy Manufacturers
of America, added: ". . . we do, however, violently and bit-
terly, and I hate to use a word quite as strong as that, oppose
the legislation the way it is currently written because frankly
we are confused. We don't quite know what it means."

But apparently Congress knew what it meant, because the
bill was passed over these objections—even though the overworked FDA will have its hands full trying to administer this
as part of the Hazardous Substances Act.

If Congress had sturdy opposition trying to push through
laws that would give the consumer half a chance for safety, it
ran into just as much, if not more, opposition in trying to get
some sanity from industry as far as flammable fabrics, blankets, curtains, paint, and other home fire hazards were con-

cerned. Tireless Senators Frank Moss and Warren Magnuson again led the fight, this time with additional and surly opposition not only from industry but from the U.S. Department of Commerce, long known as another handmaiden of the big corporations.

Not unexpectedly, the most serious concern about flammable fabrics centers on children's clothing, especially nightwear. Tragic cases of children being hideously burned through the ignition of pajamas and nightgowns are repeated with such monotonous regularity that they almost lose their shock value.

One little six-year-old girl from Ann Arbor, Michigan, got up early one morning with her father, kissed him good-bye as he left for work, then popped into bed with her mother for some moments. She then left, her mother thought, to get dressed.

Instead, she decided to go down to the kitchen, wearing her light cotton flannel pajamas, to make herself a cup of tea. She lit the left front burner of the gas stove, then reached across it to get some tea. The flame caught the right front part of the pajamas, and the pajama top turned into a torch in a matter of seconds. Hearing the child's screams, the mother rushed to the kitchen. She ripped the child's burning pajama top off, threw it in the sink, and called the doctor. He suggested wrapping cold, wet towels over the burned areas, which she did. At the hospital, where the child was rushed, second- and third-degree burns were discovered on the right side, back, chest, and upper arm. She had been wearing pajamas with the brand name of Her Majesty, made of 100-percent cotton.

In other cases, the clothing cannot be removed so quickly. One normal, healthy four-year-old boy nicked his bathrobe on the flame of a kitchen stove, and when his screams brought his mother rushing to the kitchen, she could only wrench the bathrobe off, as the flames of the pajamas enveloped the boy. Then she tried to wrap the boy in a blanket, but this failed to put the flames out. Finally, she shoved and guided the burning boy to the shower, where at last the

flames subsided. Meanwhile, the burning bathrobe had set
fire to the rug, and she had to leave the screaming child to
fight the carpet fire with pots and pans full of water. As she
did this, her feet were severely burned, as well as her hand,
all resulting from her attempts to extinguish the burning pajamas of her boy. He sustained third-degree burns over 30
percent of his body.

Fire hazards are a serious and growing situation. The
United States has *the highest per capita death rate* in the world
from fires. It is double that of Canada, four times that of
Great Britain, and six and a half times that of Japan. Over
200,000 burn cases each year are traced to fabrics. Some
3,000 of the deaths are from flaming clothing. Over 1,000
deaths come from sheets, blankets, and mattresses. And
deaths are sometimes more merciful than the agonizing injuries. Children's nightclothes account for 6,000 burn cases a
year.

There doesn't even need to be a live flame for some fabrics
to ignite. One cold morning in Milton, West Virginia, young
Scott Fugate hustled back into his house to warm up from a
cold November afternoon. He huddled near the space heater
in the living room, turning his back to it. There was no exposed flame involved. He was wearing a pile-lined coat, the
shell being 100-percent cotton corduroy. The interlining was
100-percent polyester. The inner pile was 100-percent acrylic
face with a 100-percent cotton back. If polyester is sand-
wiched in between two cotton layers, even if they have been
treated with fire-resistant chemicals, the new "sandwich" be-
haves entirely differently from either of the fabrics by itself,
according to Dr. Henry Hill, president of the Riverside Research Laboratories in Haverhill, Massachusetts.

Scott Fugate leaned against the space heater for a minute
or so, and his coat roared up in flames. He was agonizingly
burned.

This type of incident is far from uncommon. A four-year-
old girl backed up against a space heater, and her dress went
up in flames. Dr. Abraham Bergman, a pediatrician from
Seattle, treated her and hundreds of other children who will

be scarred for life from fabric burns. He has been so agonized himself by the suffering of his little patients that one time he found himself praying that one of them, who had no chance whatever to live, would die soon rather than weeks later. "How many bodies have to be stacked up before effective action is taken to prevent clothing burn injuries?" he asked. Then he added: "The textile industry, particularly those dealing in cotton, do not recognize the existence of the Flammable Fabrics Act. Their line has not changed in 10 years; namely, that a serious problem from fabric burns does not exist; that most people who get burned are careless fools who need to be educated; and that technology does not exist to treat items such as children's apparel with flame retardant finishes. Some industry spokesmen sound like they want the burned bodies piled up in front of them like cordwood before they will admit that there is even a problem."

The industry fight against the strengthening of the Flammable Fabrics Act is so typical of all industries when they are faced with consumer-protective legislation that it hardly bears repeating. Much of the fault comes from the fact that the Department of Commerce is set up to be somewhat of a sales promotion agency for all business. Warnings, labels, and retooling for safety are not great profit-making elements. Putting teeth into the act is the job of four different government agencies, and buck-passing is easy. The Commerce Department is supposed to set standards; to do this it consults with the National Advisory Council on the Flammable Fabrics Act, a council overloaded with industry representatives. One high Commerce official used to lobby for the National Cotton Council. As usual, the textile industry associations insist that voluntary standards are just the thing to solve the problem—which is tantamount to saying they'll do nothing about it.

After dragging its feet for years, the Department of Commerce finally did impose regulations to ban the sale of sleepwear for children after 1973. If a manufacturer hasn't complied by June, 1972, he must put on a label that states his garment doesn't meet with government standards. It took from 1967 until July, 1971, for the Commerce Department to get this far. Senator Moss looked on the sluggish action by the department as "too little, too late."

The parade of silent, invisible hazards doesn't stop there. Since most products are not required to be proved safe before they are put on the market, the consumer is more often than not at the mercy of the fallible and sometimes ruthless judgment of the manufacturer.

No one ever accused General Electric of deliberately producing over 150,000 color TV sets in 1966 and 1967 that would disperse deadly X rays on adults and children, who obviously would have no way of knowing they were being so exposed. But it was incumbent on the company to anticipate such a hazard and correct it before flooding the market with the sets. In its effort to correct the situation, as Ralph Nader points out, General Electric announced that only 90,000 sets were produced with this X-ray leakage. The GE announcement said the sets "may emit soft X-radiation, in excess of desirable levels." On later investigation, this "soft radiation" turned out to be some 16,000 times as powerful as the recommended safety level. Further, General Electric waited four months before admitting to the public that thousands of color TV sets were bathing their users with X rays. Meanwhile, true to the inevitable pattern, the electronic industries association pooh-poohed any idea that such a hazard could exist. If it had not been for the insistence of several New York State agencies and an exposé by the New York *Times*, no one knows how long GE would have kept the story under its hat. Radiation exposure can strike with early, acute symptoms that occur within a few hours or weeks or can have delayed effects that show up only after months or years. Often victims with acute symptoms seem healed, only to come down with leukemia later.

A medical doctor said at one time that if he could write, he'd write a story about a doctor who wanted to do away with a victim. The doctor would rent an office on the other side of the intended victim's apartment. He would then set up an X-ray machine, aim it at the wall, and dispose of his victim very handily and without any mess.

But this is taking place in reality in large cities all over the country. Hanson Blatz, director of radiation control of New York City, said: "In employing unusual techniques, it is quite possible to direct the beam at an unshielded wall and thereby expose occupants of the next room excessively. I am quite certain that we would find this in other places, like building corridors, basements and nearby sidewalks that have been found to be often momentarily subjected to relatively high intensity X-rays during the operation of nearby X-ray equipment."

Medical X rays are of deep concern to health officials. There are 17,000 medical and dental X-ray machines in New York City, and according to Hanson Blatz, most of them are twenty, thirty, and even forty years old. Most old machines do not have good aiming facilities, and rays are scattered through parts of the body that are of no diagnostic interest. The overuse of the fluoroscope is another problem. These machines expose the patient to hundreds of times as much radiation as the same examination done with an X ray.

Other radiation hazards to the general public include X-ray shoe-fitting machines that were exposed as radically dangerous years ago. Some states still permit them.

For the householder, the dangers in microwave ovens are of specific interest. Because the heating effect of the ovens is undetectable while it is in operation, the eyes, testes, gall bladder, urinary bladder, and intestines can be seriously affected. A survey by the Public Health Service revealed that twenty-five out of seventy-six microwave or "radar" ovens examined released excessive energy levels. No hazard warning labels were observed on any of the ovens. Only two of those operating the ovens had any idea that they were hazardous. Even repairmen were unaware of microwave hazards. Since most of these ovens are installed at kitchen-counter height, the eyes and upper parts of the body are particularly vulnerable to leakage from the edges of the oven door or through the open oven door. Legislation is still confused and inadequate in this field and in the whole field of radiation.

The story on detergents, phosphates, enzymes, the detergent chemical NTA (nitrilotriacetic acid), caustic soda, and just plain soap is one of the most confusing of modern times. Even the experts are baffled, although this syndrome seems to be prevalent among all the facets of foods, drugs, and cosmetics. Complicating the matter is that the problem breaks down into two departments: (1) environmental pollution, and (2) personal danger to the user. The sudden and dramatic reversal of opinion by Surgeon General Jesse L. Steinfield and FDA Commissioner Edwards to recommend a return to phosphates because of the dangers in detergents made with caustic soda seemed to bring the merry-go-round back to where it started, only to launch it off again on another senseless spin. Immediately, Steinfield and Edwards were accused of selling out to the big soap and detergent makers in their new about-face. But worse than that, the public was left reeling in confusion. There is still no clear-cut answer. Adding to the confusion was the abortive attempt of the detergent makers to replace phosphates with NTA, which turned out to be capable of producing an increase in fetal mortality in laboratory rats. One of the few sensible things the FDA seemed to do was to turn down a suspiciously generous offer from the soap and detergent industry to undertake and finance a study on whether enzyme detergents were harmful to users or to those wearing clothes laundered with the material. At least that comic-opera study was avoided. In the meantime, the National Academy of Sciences signed a contract to handle the research in February, 1971.

About the only thing a consumer can do is shrug and use as few and as little as possible of soaps and detergents until some kind of consistent pattern emerges. Meanwhile, it is safe to say that any caustic soda cleaning agent is dangerous and should be used with care. They are all either harmful to

swallow, or dangerous eye irritants, or injurious to the skin—
or all of those things together. Just a few of those named by
the FDA as having some or all of these uninviting qualities
include Miracle White, Cascade, All, Fab, Cheer, Cold
Power, Ecolo-G, and Tide XK. If you're interested in avoid-
ing phosphates, there is some slim comfort in knowing those
products that contain absolutely no amounts whatever. According to the U.S. Department of the Interior, they include:
Add-it, Culligan Soap, Diaper Sweet and Ivory Flakes in the
detergent class. In the additive class, Fels Naphtha Bar, Bora-
teem, Borax, Right Fabric Softener, and Sal Soda are simon
pure as far as being free of phosphates. In bleaches and bluing, only La France Bluing is listed as being pure. All-purpose cleaners that have no phosphates whatever are Amway
L.O.C. and 20 Mule Team Household. On the opposite end
of the spectrum, Fluffy All and Bonus are among the detergents with the highest amount of phosphates in them.

Nearly every home is a potential deathtrap, and no
amount of regulation can assure absolute safety. About all
the laws can do is reduce the hazards. Threats lurk in almost
any direction you turn in an average home.

Liquid household drain cleaners have been especially dangerous, and a rising number of serious injuries and deaths
have been caused by the ingestion of even small quantities of
these. Antidotes are useless, because destruction of the esophagus and stomach walls can set in only a few seconds after
swallowing. Charcoal briquettes might set the scene for a
pleasant party on the terrace, but their use indoors or in
tents, trailers, automobiles, or boats have produced thirty-
one fatalities in recent years from the carbon monoxide they
give off. Many batches of Mexican and other lead-filled pottery still continue to create lead poisoning. Even mild acid
solutions used in the vessels leach out the lead and free it.
Twenty-six out of twenty-eight samples of Mexican pottery
tested by the FDA contained various amounts of lead
leached from the glaze. It seems that the rough or dull glaze
gives off the most lead in such circumstances. What makes it

difficult for the consumer is that these products may or may not be marked as of Mexican origin, or whatever other country that may be involved.

Lead paint continues to plague the market, with one survey revealing that 10 percent of the paint offered for sale in New York City sold for interior use contains more lead than is allowed by law. The survey was prompted by the deaths of a leopard and several other animals in the Staten Island Zoo after chewing on the paint used there. Meanwhile, the number of slum children in New York coming down with lead poisoning from chewing on painted surfaces rose 300 percent from 1969 to 1970.

Nearly 120,000 Americans are injured each year by unsafe lenses in eyeglasses. Twenty thousand of these are schoolchildren. All of this has led to the FDA announcement in September, 1970, that eyeglasses and sunglasses shall be made from impact-resistant material. Processes to make lenses of this sort have been available for years. The delay in providing this protection for so long is hard to explain.

The discovery that youngsters, especially in the eleven- to fifteen-year-old group, were spraying aerosol fumes into paper bags and inhaling them to get "high" added one more concern to the growing household hazard picture. It doesn't matter what the product is—hair spray, deodorant, household cleaner—it is the hydrocarbon or fluorocarbon propellant (Freon is the best-known trade name) that is the attraction. The FDA figures showed that four youthful deaths a month were reported. Death comes quick and sudden, from either single or multiple use, and once the reaction sets in, damage to the heart is irreversible.

Even more tragic than this intentional abuse of aerosol products is the disease that forms in the fibrous tissues of the lung caused by unintentional inhalation of aerosol products. Two female roommates came down with the disease after using the same spray deodorant over a period of time. One felt strangled and developed a cough after each use; the other found her endurance lagging precipitously.

A team of Army doctors at the Fitzsimmons General Hospital in Denver followed up with a study of ten young men using the same spray, plus one who used another brand. They came down with similar symptoms. Guinea pigs exposed to the same sprays promptly developed lung lesions.*

Aerosol manufacturers immediately began giving lip service about combating these dangers. The comment of the year came from B. J. Burkett, public relations manager for the Freon Division of Du Pont de Nemours & Company. "They're really trying awfully hard," he said of the Inter-Industry Committee on Aerosol Use. But when it came to putting label warnings on the can or bringing back the old skull-and-crossbones symbol, the manufacturers were less than enthusiastic.

Carter-Wallace finally decided to add labels to its Arrid and Easy Day deodorants with the line: "Warning: Avoid excessive inhalation which may be harmful." Again, a sentence that has impact and meaning, such as "Inhaling this spray can kill you," was neatly avoided.

Industry's skill in writing warnings in such a way that they sound like an invitation to a debutante party has been developed into a fine art. Phrases like "soft X-radiation," "excess of desirable levels," and the use of the word "may" instead of "will" are all the result of long corporation committee meetings that will go on for hours looking for euphemistic adjectives to cover up the blunt, direct terms that these warnings should carry with them.

* Several cases of pneumonia from hair sprays have been recorded in the *New England Journal of Medicine*. Further concern has been expressed by some doctors and FDA officials about the chemicals used in permanents. Widespread opinion is that both these areas need further investigation.

14

Over the Counter, and Over the Skin

A NURSE who lives in the Washington, D.C., area treated herself to a new look by dyeing her hair with a Clairol hair dye and was pleased with the results. It wasn't long, however, before she began to notice that her urine had turned black. Cautiously, she tried the same treatment later, with the same result. She made a careful study of the label, but nowhere could she find the full chemical ingredients of the product listed on the package.

She was not alone. FDA researchers received several complaints from others who had used Clairol's Silk and Silver and Loving Care that their urine had turned black after using them. When the skins of laboratory mice were painted with the products, the urine of the mice turned black consistently after the application. Neither the FDA nor the Clairol company could find what was causing the reaction, and after a series of tests, the research activity was tabled in favor of more pressing problems. Clairol protested that their research found that the products were safe and has continued to produce them with the ingredients—whatever they are, because Clairol isn't telling—unchanged. Since cosmetic and toiletry manufacturers enjoy the legal privilege of putting whatever they want into a product, except specific color additives, both the public and the FDA seldom know what a cosmetic contains, and there's no legal way to do anything about it. As with therapeutic devices, the only recourse the government has is the seizure of a single shipment at a time and long, endless legal battles if something shows up to be dangerous.

Cosmetics are part of the vast consumer jungle known as the over-the-counter market. In addition to cosmetics, it includes the old-fashioned patent medicines, which is a more graphic description of what the manufacturers like to call "proprietary" drugs. (Many of them are worthless nostrums. Estimates are that 85 percent of them show no adequate evidence of being effective.) Diet and reducing pills, toiletries, dentifrices, soaps and shampoos, and other products consistently emerge as being of dubious or no value. The public spends about $2.5 billion a year on at least 100,000 different kinds of over-the-counter drugs. Aspirin production alone comes to 18,000 tons each year, or enough for 225 tablets for each person in the United States. The cosmetic industry takes in about $6 billion annually.

The FDA efforts to harness the $6-billion cosmetic business are more than pinched by the budget allocation of the department that handles this end of the regulations. In a recent year, the FDA cosmetic-control budget was 1/6,000th of the cosmetics dollar volume and less than 1½ percent of the FDA manpower and dollar budget. Since the cosmetics area is one where a great many potential time bombs exist, two steps are obligatory for some semblance of rational control: (1) laws requiring the premarket screening of new products, (2) the full disclosure of the manufacturer's complaint file to the FDA.

Dr. Jacqueline Verrett, the outspoken FDA scientist, is concerned about the loose laws that govern the entire cosmetic and toiletry industry. "Cosmetics are a total disaster area," she says. "Lipstick dyes are far from being properly tested, yet they're eaten by women as constantly as children eat lollipops. Many cosmetics pose a serious dermal problem. We don't have the faintest idea about most of the formulas used by the cosmetic manufacturers. We know they're using some coal-tar dyes—but the FDA has no control over how they put these mixtures together, or what's in them besides coal tar. One company wanted to use irradiation to sterilize its eye shadow. Another disaster, if permitted. I read one cosmetic formula fast, and found that half the materials used were carcinogenic. Hair dyes—they're absorbed through the scalp and into the system. Very little is known about what happens here."

The root of the hair dye problem seems to lie in a chemical known as 2,4-TDA, a part of the hair dye component but not a hair dye itself. Coal-tar dyes were banned as long ago as 1938, but the cosmetic industry managed to slip a loophole in the laws indicating that they could be used in hair dyes if a warning were put on the label indicating that a "patch test" should be made on the skin before using. Just how many women take this trouble, which involves twenty-four hours, is uncertain.

In early 1971, a major hair dye study concentrating on 2,4-TDA was still continuing, and results were not expected for at least a year. Meanwhile, there were clear and definite things known about the chemical, the principal one being that it definitely produced cancer when injected under the skin of laboratory animals. Clairol is not the only firm to use the chemical. Breck, Revlon, Toni, and others have used it regularly for a total of forty-three different brands.

Although tests on laboratory animals do not necessarily reflect what might happen in the human system, most scientists agree that positive findings in animal tests simply *cannot* be ignored. The carcinogenic properties of 2,4-TDA have for all practical purposes been ignored since 1949, when the initial cancer-producing findings were made. In the mid-sixties, the FDA determined that 2,4-TDA was present in hair dyes, but practically nothing was done about it. The cancer potential is joined by other threats in the use of hair dyes. The scalp can break out unpredictably with rashes, sores, or swellings.

Mercury in fish and in the environment is bad enough, but this heavy metal has been deliberately pumped into all kinds of cosmetics in far larger doses than that found in tuna fish—just about twenty times as much, to be exact. Since the ingredients of cosmetics are not generally known, no one can tell what products contain mercury or not. Creams, lotions, hair preparations, and facial makeup are found to be the most likely products containing mercury, placed there by the manufacturers as a preservative. FDA scientists are most concerned about its use in body lotions, since they are applied to large areas of the skin.

Since the mercury problem elsewhere may have serious implications, the additional load of mercury through its use in cosmetics compounds the felony. This metal is absorbed through the skin and stored in the kidneys. Pressed for an answer about mercury, an industry representative admitted that it has been widely used to prevent contamination of cosmetics by microorganisms, but that its use was on the way out. Meanwhile the manufacturers' group refused to give the FDA a list of which products contained mercury and how much. As Ron Nessen, of NBC-TV, pointed out, FDA scientists found they had to go down to the corner drugstore and buy the cosmetics they wanted to test, a technique known as market-basket research. Meanwhile, the consumer who goes to the drugstore has no idea which cosmetics have mercury preservatives in them, how much is in them, or how harmful they might be to her. In foods, no tolerance level for mercury is permitted, except for the provisional allowance with tuna of .05 parts per million.

Other metals linger ominously in cosmetics, among them being zinc (in antidandruff preparations) and lead (in hair-coloring preparations). Although this use of lead has been cleared by the FDA in color additives, it is only deemed provisionally safe. There is a definite and certain danger, however, in the unlikely chance that you would use the hair preparation and lick your fingers afterward.

The colors used in lipsticks are supposed to be cleared under the color additives law and therefore safe, although there are many qualified experts who disagree that this is adequate protection. Most lipsticks are made up of castor oil, perfume, flavoring, beeswax, and added color. A good many of these colors have been delisted in the past, but only after long periods of considerable use. Still, many lipstick ingredients remain trade secrets, and therein lies the rub.

Not even certified colors are allowed in products used around the eyes, but inorganic chemicals such as iron oxides, chrome oxides, and a few naturally derived organics are used. Not harmful but rather squirmy to think about is that one basic ingredient of eye shadow is carmine, which is made up of finely ground cochineal bugs, packed together at the rate of 70,000 insects per pound.

A main and constant problem across the board in cosmetics is contamination of microorganisms—a special nightmare for eye specialists who constantly run into patients with infections resulting from cosmetics. The eyes are especially vulnerable, in contrast to the skin, although any breaks in the skin offer a good chance of infection from contamination. *Pseudomonas* contamination of eye shadow, mascara, eye lotions, or drops can be very serious. Staph infection is not uncommon from the use of cosmetics. Conditions like these arise often from borrowing or trading off cosmetics—a fairly common practice among women who like to try different kinds.

Recalls of cosmetic products are frequent. Roux Laboratories had its lash and brow tint recalled at one time because its ingredients, silver sulfate, silver nitrate, and pyrogallol, were found to be unsafe. Some of Max Factor's Tried and True Proteined Hair Conditioner was also found by the FDA not to live up to its name. A shipment of this product was found to contain uninvited mold. Elizabeth Arden's Hand Lotion June Geranium was recalled in one case because of bacterial contamination. Avon's Topaze Cologne Mist met the same fate because the product contained an unacceptable color agent, and another batch of the same product was found to be adulterated.

Exorbitantly expensive facial creams are considered to be no more effective than ordinary-priced products as far as keeping the skin young and fresh. A cream known as Irma Shorell Contour/35 was offered to the unsuspecting public at $27.50 a jar, with the promise that it would "rejuvenate and restore youth to the skin, is equivalent and may be used instead of surgical face lifting, and will have a permanent or lasting effect." The FTC (Federal Trade Commission) clamped down briskly, and the company promised not to be so extravagant in its claims in the future. In addition, the FDA got after their exorbitantly priced item because the claims made the product a drug rather than a cosmetic.

Consumer Reports gives all creams and lotions a rough time as far as their claims are concerned. The constant parade of phrases like "warding off wrinkles" or "skin penetrants" are just so much verbiage, and soap and water can probably do just as good a job, according to their surveys. The FTC recently had to get after the way Hazel Bishop was advertising its Sudden Change. The company had retouched its "before and after" pictures.

The FTC reports trouble with bleaching creams, which have habitually contained mercury as a preservative. Nitrates and borates are used in some skin creams for the same purpose, and both are injurious to the liver and kidneys and may be cancer-producing.

Hormone cream safety depends on how much of the hormones are absorbed. Ordinary use has not raised any FDA eyebrows, but any inordinate use ought to be under a doctor's care and recommendation.

There is no such thing as a benefit-to-risk ratio in cosmetics. They *must* be safe, and the consumer has a right to know what's in the products she is buying. As long as cosmetic makers are not legally obligated to tell the public or the FDA what is in the product, or as long as they don't have to show proof that they are safe before marketing, there is bound to be trouble lurking throughout the entire industry.

The same problem applies as far as toiletries and dentifrice products are concerned. The mouthwash racket—and that is exactly the correct word for it—has been going on for so many years that the consumer is numb to it.

The Warner-Lambert pharmaceutical kingdom is the corporation that has the questionable honor of bringing to the public the next-to-worthless mouthwash known as Listerine.

This antediluvian product has been hanging around for decades and was the subject of major criticism some forty years ago in Kallet and Schlink's *100,000,000 Guinea Pigs.*

Back in 1933, the authors wrote: "Ranked in order of efficiency in killing the four test organisms, Listerine, most blatantly advertised and one of the most widely sold of antiseptics, was fifth from the bottom of the list, being rated lowest among the popular proprietary antiseptics tested. It failed to kill *bacillus pyocyaneus* and *staphylococcus aureus* in four different tests even after three hours. In one test, it killed *bacillus subtilis* only after more than 30 minutes of contact, failing to kill it in three other tests after three hours. . . ."

Yet today, in the 1970's, a recent Warner-Lambert annual report states: "Listerine, the division's leading product, increased its unit dollar sale and share of the market . . . a product found effective by consumers over the past 80 years." The report did not explain what laboratory tests the average consumer had at his command to prove the mouthwash effective. Certainly not scientific appraisals.

What does the final report of the National Academy of Sciences say not just about Listerine but about *all* mouthwashes? It states: "There is no convincing evidence that any medicated mouthwash, used as a part of a daily hygiene regimen, has therapeutic advantage over a physiologic saline solution *or even water.*" (Italics added.)

There are many other interesting things in this portion of the NAS final report. In addition to stating that without exception there is no mouthwash on the market that meets the acceptance standards outlined by the Council of Dental Therapeutics, it adds that any commercial mouthwash can upset the normal oral flora, and that "the desirability of permitting these products to be sold directly to the public is questionable." The NAS report was the basis for the FDA to take action to ban claims on many leading brands of mouthwashes, including Lever Brothers' Pepsodent Mouthwash; Richardson-Merrell's Cepacol; and Johnson & Johnson's Micrin Oral Antiseptic. The action will be extended for other mouthwashes currently marketed.

Similar FDA action against ten widely sold toothpastes as a result of the NAS final report on drug efficacy was the reason Brisk, Colgate Chlorophyll Toothpaste with Gardol, Colgate Dental Cream with Gardol, Kolynos Fluoride Toothpaste, and Amm-i-Dent toothpaste were cited as being ineffective. Other citations will follow; this is preliminary.

Much has been said about stannous fluoride in toothpaste and its ability to reduce cavities. But a 1969 British study showed that the same ingredient was clearly responsible for a brown-and-black staining of the teeth. Stannous flouride is what Crest toothpaste brags about as its most active ingredient, under the trade name Fluoristan. A Crest commercial showing a happy kid yelling, "Our group had twenty percent more brown stains!" is yet to be heard.

If the toothpastes and mouthwashes are having a rough time, Dr. West's Germ Fighter toothbrush was not faring any better. The Chemway Corporation, makers of the brush, offered this sort of enlightening advertising about the product:

> Citizens, throw away your toothbrushes. They're crawling with germs, things like Staphylococcus Aureus and Streptococcus Pyogenes. As soon as you crack a toothbrush out of its plastic case, the collection starts. And by the time you brush a few times, there may be millions of germs. . . . Buy the Germ Fighter toothbrush by Dr. West's. It's treated with a compound that inhibits the growth of germs at least four months.

The FTC took a dimmer view of the situation. Its complaint stated very directly: "In truth and in fact, the antibacterial property of Dr. West's Germ Fighter toothbrush is of no medical significance in killing germs likely to cause infectious diseases of the oral cavity, and use of such product has no significant effect in the mitigation or prevention of infectious diseases of the oral cavity." Further, the Dr. West company had saturated the brush and handle with a mercury compound that could easily be leached off and ingested during normal brushing—another mercury threat to add to the growing list. If you haven't seen much Dr. West's tooth-brush advertising around lately, it may be because the FTC ordered the company to devote at least one-quarter of any ads it may run to stating that the FTC has alleged that the company made false assertions in its previous advertising.

Advertising chicanery is so constant that the consumer often throws up his hands and gives in to it out of sheer fatigue. Bristol-Myers, constantly popping up with problems for the FDA or the FTC, tried a neat little trick with Dry Ban, one of its spray antiperspirants. Its agency, Ogilvy & Mather, engineered a series of five commercials titled "Rusty Rev," "Show UP," "Dry Manhattan," "Spotty Perform-ance," and "Glasses."

During these tense dramas dredged out of Madison Ave-nue's finest talents, we see Dry Ban and another "leading spray" sprayed onto a dark surface. The competing spray is white and thick, but not Dry Ban. It looks so clear and dry that you've got to gasp in admiration. The announcer, of course, has to put his benediction on the matter by asking voice-over: "Which do you prefer?"

A similar drama takes place in another of the commer-cials. This time it's two girls in an elevator, one of whom does the same trick on a pair of eyeglass lenses. One of the girls, a master of witty rhetoric, says: "I see the difference!" And the announcer comes in to top this off with: "Clear Dry Ban helps keep you feeling clean and dry."

The FTC looked at the commercials in a different light. It ordered Bristol-Myers to stop this kind of nonsense, since not only was there no product superiority demonstrated here, but Dry Ban isn't a dry spray at all, and when it does dry out, it leaves a visible residue. The battle against the inanity of tele-vision commercials has been going on since television began. There is no real safety issue at stake with Dry Ban, but what advertisers are doing with this they are doing with medicines and preparations that seriously involve the health and safety of the entire family.

If you pick up an aerosol container of Gillette's The Hot

One Self Heating Shave Cream, you will notice that the instructions say to point the nozzle straight down. It further says never to actuate the valve with nozzle pointing up and not to use if the lather appears watery or soupy. In case itching or irritation develop, you are to discontinue use immediately.

The reason for this lies in the fact that self-heating aerosol products have some tricky problems with dispensing technique, according to *Chemical Week*. A spokesman for the company that makes the valve assembly for this kind of dispenser said:

> Some skin irritation problems have arisen because of improper concentrations of chemicals. An excess of the 10 per cent peroxide could well burn the skin. If the valve is operated at the normal angle, the peroxide-sulfite ratio works out properly. But if the operating angle is distorted, so is the ratio. For example, if the valve is just cracked—"teased"—you'll wind up with a handful of peroxide from the pouch. Or if you "blast" the valve, holding it wide open, you'll get an excess of sulfite, which may give off a foul odor on contact with the skin.

The problem is that very few shavers take the time to read the instructions carefully. Consequently, their skin may be dosed regularly with either sulfite or peroxide, and a rash may develop.

A curious thing happened with Pfizer's product called Un-Burn, advertised by the company for relief of sunburn pain. The FTC filed a complaint that Pfizer's advertisements falsely implied that adequate and well-controlled scientific tests were made before the product was marketed. However, an FTC hearing examiner found in a preliminary decision that the active ingredients, benzocaine and menthol, had been in successful use for many years, and therefore the charges were dismissed.

What were not brought up, however, were the findings of the National Academy of Sciences review of this sort of product, relating to the use of benzocaine. The NAS report said: "Benzocaine is a notorious sensitizer which should be avoided by individuals with dermatitis of the hands from any cause." In addition the NAS dermatology panel said:

> In summary, topical anesthetics [those used on skin to relieve pain] appear to be effective when applied to mucous membranes or damaged skin. Their effectiveness in skin conditions with an intact epidermis remains to be shown. However, it is under the same conditions where these agents are effective (applications to mucous membranes and damaged skin) that they are most likely to produce toxic or hypersensitivity reactions. . . . Accepting the fact that the anesthetic ointments are effective in the proper circumstances, one may raise the question of their over-the-counter [versus prescription only] status due particularly to their sensitizing effects.

In other words, products containing benzocaine and many other local anesthetic components are a potential hazard, and there is a question mark in the minds of the NAS scientists as to whether this sort of compound should remain available without prescription. Meanwhile, it would not hurt a consumer to exercise caution in using any anesthetic ointment.

When the problem came up with the bubble bath delights for children, there was a very weak label warning parents that such products as Gold Seal's Mr. Bubble, Purex's Flintstones, and Bubble Club Fun Bath were dangerous to children. Complaints have been received by the FDA that some bubble bath products could lead to bacterial infections of the urinary tract, general skin irritation, and damage to the genitalia.

The difficult part of this sort of situation in the soap-and-cosmetics area is, of course, that there is no legislation for pretesting, and the FDA cannot legally ban the sale of a product that produces this kind of reaction. Even though both companies agreed to reformulate the products, it is incredible that a manufacturer would offer an item that would obviously have the potential, at least, of injuring children. The launching of any product for children certainly requires extreme caution before putting it on the market. An ironic part about this incident is that after the FDA rapped both companies on the knuckles, a number of stores in the Washington area disposed of the supplies they had on hand by marking the products down in price, according to reporter Elizabeth Shelton, in the Washington *Post.*

Meanwhile, the FDA is now following through on a check of all bubble bath products on the market with a component called alkyl aryl sulfonate as the suspected irritant. And, with the lack of labeling laws, who knows what's in a product? The FDA has nothing to report on the use of regular detergents in the bathtub, which are sometimes used by adults and children to prevent the classic ring around the tub. Common sense would indicate caution.

Action by the FDA is also being contemplated against eye-irritating shampoos, the result of the discovery that Consolidated Royal's castile shampoo produced eye injuries in test animals. Also under sharp suspicion is the antidandruff agent used in Head and Shoulders and Breck One. Proposed future plans are tests on human volunteers for all these products. One of the major problems with shampoos has been those purporting to prevent any stinging of the eyes, a regular complaint of children when their hair is being washed. The only catch to the trick of making non-eye-stinging shampoos is that a local anesthetic is used, which might be very convenient for removing the sting but extremely dangerous for a youngster's—or adult's—eyes.

The hexachlorophene story built up slowly. Since the first FDA announcement about it, the word going around the cosmetic and toiletry industry was that practically every company was searching frantically for a substitute for hexachlorophene because so many items have been intentionally riddled with the substance. The irony of this chemical, which is first cousin to the deadly Vietnam herbicide 2,4,5-T, is that it has been such a featured sales hook on everything from Dial soap to mouthwashes, toothpastes, deodorants, medicated talcs, feminine sprays, hospital soaps and, especially, cosmetics. New stories are breaking constantly on its dangers, and just how the sales promotion geniuses will twist the sales and advertising approach will be interesting. Undoubtedly, there will be a major campaign with headlines reading: "New! Dial Soap's Fresh Improved Formula Brings You Greater Protection with Greater Safety than Ever Before!" It's almost a sure bet that very little will be said about hexachlorophene and its quiet demise. Advertising agencies in situations like this find an opportunity to really display their genius, like the copywriter's gag in trying to devise a headline on how to sell a secondhand pencil that had lost its eraser. The winning headline was: PRETESTED PENCIL—ABSOLUTELY LATEX-FREE!

Confident of the germicidal properties of hexachlorophene, mothers have been liberally soaking, dousing, and smearing their infants with pHisoHex, Johnson & Johnson First Aid Cream, baby powders, and other products, secure in their feeling that they couldn't be doing more for the protection of their offspring. Two journalists, one in Asia and the other in Africa, used almost nothing but pHisoHex for "dry" bathing, principally because many of the areas they were in had nothing but a highly impure water supply.

The fact that several babies have gone into convulsions after being bathed with a hexachlorophene soap and that one of the journalists came down with a year-long severe lesion of the scrotum that resisted all treatment seemed to tie in with some tests conducted at the government's Communicable Disease Center (CDC) in Atlanta. The tests, oddly enough, arose out of experiments designed to examine the chemical for its usefulness as a pesticide. Dr. Renate Kimbrough, of the CDC, found that it produced definite brain damage to rats at very low feeding levels. In addition, its use in some burn cases on humans had demonstrated the same sort of damage to the brain, as the patients went into convulsions and died as a result. Further studies were beginning to show that hexachlorophene proved to be teratogenetic—causing abnormalities in animal offspring.

All of this momentum gathered quietly, the innocent fluffy clouds that suddenly form into a thunderhead. Random samples of people using a soap, mouthwash, or cosmetic containing hexachlorophene began to show deposits of the chemical in the bloodstream and fatty tissues after just three weeks of normal use. One FDA scientist, a volunteer guinea pig using Dial soap for some of the tests, said: "I have to admit I feel somewhat uncomfortable about all this."

The feminine hygiene sprays containing hexachlorophene are particularly suspect because of the direct contact with the mucous membranes more sensitive than the scrotum or penis, and they carry the added danger of exposing the tissues to excessive cooling from the aerosol spray and its freon gases.

What makes the situation more than a simple concern is that the use of hexachlorophene has been growing and compounding itself by proliferation in many products where it would be of absolutely no value to the consumer, even if it were safe. The shadows of the carbon tet fiasco seem to lurk here. Manufacturers found some kind of magic in stamping CONTAINS HEXACHLOROPHENE on their labels and packages, as if it were the panacea of all time. Nowhere could you find mention that it was dangerous, even before the new tests were beginning to show lethal possibilities. Even the mild warning that it must be thoroughly washed off after use was usually ignored.

Its use in wounds has now become cause for alarm, according to the experts, and the larger the wound, the more dangerous the application. By February, 1971, a stack of new reports of the Center for Communicable Diseases on its dangers had not yet been published. The larger the area of skin exposed, the more likelihood of absorption into the bloodstream—yet the babies who had been bathed from head to toe with pHisoHex (with a high 3-percent content) are uncountable. And even though scientists had known for years that hexachlorophene is a poison to the central nervous system, old-style methodology had no way of discerning the systemic absorption of the chemical into the bloodstream. The product was used freely in water for cattle to prevent liver fluke, and in Europe it was added as a safeguard for children's drinking water.

Puzzling is the laboratory evidence in animals showing that the product might have the possibility of creating *reversible* brain damage. All prior medical data have shown that the destruction of brain cells or damage to the brain cells is permanent; it cannot be reversed.

As the evidence built up, the question of what to do about the situation pressed hard on the FDA. Here was a popular product, used mainly on the surface of the skin, that was capable of producing serious systemic damage, even death and convulsions. On the other hand, the assembling of the evidence, the appraisal of it, and the ultimate conclusions from it might not hold up in court and thus damage the case for future seizures of any products containing the substance.

A cautious press release was prepared, not issued until April 1, 1971, which reflected practically none of the anxiety boiling beneath the surface calm of the agency. It read:

PRESS RESPONSE STATEMENT

Hexachlorophene has been used extensively in the past 20 years as an antiseptic for application to the skin and as a fungicide and bactericide for agricultural products. In addition to usage in soaps and solutions, it has also been employed in recent years as a constituent of deodorants, anti-perspirants and feminine hygiene products, mouthwashes, and toothpastes. Current studies by Dr. Francis Marzulli, FDA toxicologist, and by outside investigators are under way to extend our knowledge of the behavior of hexachlorophene under various conditions of usage. That the substance has toxic qualities is well-known; without such qualities hexachlorophene would not be effective as an antiseptic. Precautions stated on all labels of concentrated solutions of hexachlorophene should be carefully observed at all times. Rinsing is advised after any application and should be particularly thorough when dealing with wounds and extensive burns. At this time and on the basis of information now available, FDA plans no regulatory action concerning hexachlorophene.

There were many scientists around the FDA who thought this release was a masterpiece of understatement. One outspoken FDA scientist said: "How can we continue permitting the use of this hazard just for the sake of the empires built on it? We know that it's absorbed through the skin. We know it can cause systemic damage in humans, even in dilute solutions. We know that when other impurities are added to it, its potency is enhanced. We know what it does to the central nervous system and brains of laboratory animals. Before the evidence mounted up, there may have been some excuse for it in controlled medical situations. As for its use in cosmetics, it should have been thrown out years ago. And what about the long term, long range use? Do people have to fall over dead before we take action?"

Some of the people who were falling over in a dead faint, at least, were the top executives of Armour-Dial, the makers of Dial soap. In April, 1971, they scurried with little ceremony to the FDA offices, but what was said in their meeting with the equally top brass of the FDA never leaked out. One major concern of everybody connected with the use of the chemical was whether it resided in human fat with the tenacity of DDT. Another question bound to confuse the issue was whether all the myriad products boasting of their use of hexachlorophene were soaps, cosmetics, mouthwashes, deodorants, toothpastes—or were they drugs?

This is a puzzling, gray area. It is important, because if the product were to be considered a drug, then all the ingredients would have to be listed on the label or package, a fate that the cosmetic and over-the-counter toilet goods producers would consider worse than death. They had escaped this requirement during all the various and multitudinous amendments to the Food, Drug, and Cosmetic Act that were enacted all through the fifties and sixties. As cosmetics or toilet goods, products need no FDA blessing—except for color additives—before being put on the market, and the burden of proof falls on the FDA through long and costly litigation.

Because hexachlorophene has been practically the emperor of all over-the-counter toilet goods, to say nothing of its almost universal use in hospitals and doctors' offices in the form of pHisoHex, the liquid skin cleaner, the importance of this gradually unveiling horror story cannot be underestimated. Almost everyone in the country has been exposed to hexachlorophene in one way or another.

There had been so much talk and so little action by the FDA in clamping down on the use of this chemical, known also as G-11, that needless exposure by infants and adults continued all through 1971, while the dangers became more and more obvious.

The growing concern about the chemical was shoved into a very mild, unnoticed limelight on March 29, 1971, when August Curley and Robert Hawk, research chemists of the Environmental Protection Agency, revealed that hexachlorophene had caused cerebral swelling and brain damage in rats and was found in the blood of human beings, because the chemical had penetrated directly through normal, healthy skin.

Several small stories appeared in the press about this, and as a result the FDA issued its cautious and soft-pedaled warning on April 1.

Back in 1959, over a decade before any of the public heard any noise about this threat to life and limb, a newborn infant was brought home from the hospital, and his mother treated him to a rich pHisoHex (3 percent hexachlorophene) lotion after his bath. After four days, the baby's buttocks and face were covered with ugly sores, and his arms, legs, and face began a slight, uncontrollable twitching. Slowly over the days, the twitching became more pronounced and then turned into full-scale convulsions.

When the baby reached the hospital on his eleventh day, his skin was red all over, his arms and legs were jerking violently, and his face was still twitching. His eyes were moving wildly in their sockets, a condition known as roving nystagmus. The left side of his face was paralyzed. With the pHiso-Hex lotion discontinued, the baby slowly began to improve, and he survived. All these symptoms were the result of direct absorption through the originally normal, healthy skin of the infant. A mild warning on the pHisoHex container indicated that the fluid should be thoroughly rinsed off. It is in small type and unlikely to be read or seen by a large percentage of busy mothers. A statement like this would be more appropriate: UNLESS YOU RINSE THIS OFF, YOU OR YOUR BABY CAN GO INTO CONVULSIONS. HEXACHLOROPHENE CAN BUILD UP IN YOUR BLOOD. BRAIN LESIONS AND CEREBRAL SWELLINGS HAVE OCCURRED ON THE SKIN OF LABORATORY RATS FROM SURFACE USE ON INTACT SKIN. ACCIDENTAL SWALLOWING' OF pHISOHEX CAN KILL YOU.

At this writing, the subsidiary of Sterling Drug, makers of pHisoHex, aren't inclined to include something like this in the warning. The danger of swallowing the product is unquestioned. Back in 1963, a six-year-old retarded child drank about two shot glasses full of pHisoHex and was dead nine hours later. One very real problem with pHisoHex is that it looks much like milk of magnesia and has often been taken by mistake as such. In 1966, still long before any of this news leaked out publicly, a seventeen-day-old infant was accidentally given hexachlorophene orally. Within four days, the baby's skull began bulging strangely, his extremities began having spasms, and his face, too, began twitching. His head thrashed back and forth, and his lips continuously sucked unnaturally. He eventually recovered, but the story was never included in any of Sterling Drug's promotional literature or on the pHisoHex label.

In 1968 a scientist named D. L. Larson reported in the American Hospitals Association journal that a 3-percent solution of hexachlorophene—the amount found in pHisoHex, passed easily through burn wounds into the bloodstream, and convulsions resulted in both children and adults. Some patients developed stupor, coma, confusion, muscle twitching, and cerebral edema.

Even mild solutions of hexachlorophene (Dial soap has 1 percent, and use of this soap has built up levels in the blood of persons using it over a period of time) leave their marks. Back in 1961, again almost a decade before anyone began seriously questioning all this, a scientific team headed by V. D. Newcomer found that a group of patients developed an ugly melanosis of the face called chloasma from various cosmetics they were using. The only thing common among these cosmetics was hexachlorophene. In the same year, one team of doctors treated twelve cases of "severe, painful dermatitis" of the scrotum, each of which had developed from the use of pHisoHex. In 1967, another scientific team, headed by F. E. Carroll, reported in a leading obstetrics journal that the chemical was easily absorbed through intact skin, and in the same year two other scientists found that hexachlorophene remained on the skin after bathing in a very weak solution of it. They also found that even after rinsing with water and sponging with alcohol, a residue was left on the skin.

The vaginal spray problem is more serious than just the harm to the vaginal tissues. A new study indicates that the use of these sprays by a mother may contribute higher blood levels in the newborn child.

Johnson & Johnson (Vespre and Naturally Feminine sprays) and Alberto-Culver (FDS spray) were incensed when the FDA finally got around to its belated firm warning in December, 1971. Both companies protested such an action against their pet products endowed with as many flavors as Jell-O. Dr. Martin L. Stone, chairman of the Department of Obstetrics of the New York Medical College, told New York *Times* reporter Grace Lichtenstein: "The sprays are sort of like pouring perfume in the area. I'd rather see the patient bathe."

Since infants and children are so vulnerable to the chemical, it is hard to understand why it has been almost a universal practice in hospitals to continually bathe newborn babies with it. While pHisoHex is effective as a preventive against staph infections, the question of benefit-to-risk ratio can be sharply questioned except in emergency situations. The British medical journal *Lancet* reported that among all babies studied in a recent test, most of them had higher levels of hexachlorophene in their blood on the day they left the hospital than on the first days of being bathed with the solution. In 1968 the skins of rats were exposed to burns and treated with hexachlorophene. All of the rats died in from two to fifteen days.

In the face of all this easily available and carefully documented scientific material, the mild FDA warning did not go out until April, 1971—and even then no immediate action was taken against Dial, pHisoHex, or any of the hundreds of other over-the-counter products using the chemical. And what happened between April, 1971, and the rest of the year? The FDA reported "continuing studies" are "currently under way." But where was the action? The usually reliable and objective news journal of the cosmetic and toiletry industry known as the Pink Sheet (also known as *F-D-C Reports*) stated on October 4, 1971—seven months after publicity started breaking—that the "FDA is taking a new and intense look at hexachlorophene to determine whether the scientific evidence, which has been building up in the past few years, requires some form of new regulatory action on HCP [hexachlorophene] products, particularly in the cosmetics area where safety is evaluated in more absolute terms than it is in the drug field."

A new and intense look? The agency had announced that back in April.

In the meantime, what has been the general attitude of the industry through all this? For one thing, the major supplier of hexachlorophene, the Givaudan Corporation, has been advertising with full-page ads in the trade journals for the benefit of cosmetic and toiletry manufacturers who are using so much of the chemical in their products with copy like this:

> When you buy G-11 (Hexachlorophene U.S.P.), there's no escaping this fact: You know well what you're getting. G-11 has been proven effective in thousands of tests around the world. . . .
>
> G-11 has been proven safe in every conceivable product. From soaps to shoe linings. Antiseptics to toothpastes. Through over 20 years of actual use, G-11 has been proven a moving force in the market place. The public knows it. Likes it. Trusts it . . . .

Not one word about the babies and burn victims in convulsions, the ugly melanosis, or even that rats died within fifteen days. And a spokesman for the Sterling Drug subsidiary that makes pHisoHex summed up his case very neatly, as if he never even read the mild FDA warning, to say nothing of the long and careful medical studies:

"PHisoHex has been used by millions of people of all ages in and out of hospitals and all over the world without harmful effects."

15

The Medicine Men

CONSENSUS among those who are concerned about the rising drug culture is that over-the-counter drug advertising on television and in magazines is totally out of control. A four-year-old child recently tried to sell his grandmother on taking Compoz when she complained about being unable to sleep. "Mood" drugs available without a prescription are of special interest. Here the advertising is most blatant, creating a dependency of both adults and children that reaches in extent far beyond the overprescribing of tranquilizers and sedatives by the physician.

Dr. William Beaver, professor of pharmacology at the George Washington University School of Medicine, tells the story of how he was called in as a consultant to an advertising agency to advise them about a new pain-killer that was being prepared for the market. But in this case, the pharmaceutical company had not researched and developed the product. They had asked the advertising agency to think up a good advertising campaign, notify the company what type of product would sell best, and the company in turn would come up with a magic nostrum to match the advertising campaign. Dr. Beaver could be nothing but negative about this idea and withdrew from the project.

Television commercials are carefully structured works of dubious art. The best technicians in the business are hired as architects for these consumer persuaders, and they can tamper so skillfully with your unconscious that you will probably find yourself buying something you didn't want or need in order to alleviate some health problem you don't have. The employment of surface drama or comedy is a baited hook in order to suck the viewer into acceptance of a "unique" benefit that the product on the screen can offer. For the most part this benefit is entirely imaginary. With adults falling for this carefully engineered impetus to the sweeping pill culture of the country, small children naturally fall in line, and older children are able to jump off on the illicit drug springboard as a natural and easy step.

One interesting phenomenon is the new trend of pawning off analgesics—pain-killers—as mood drugs to cope with all the problems of modern life. Aspirin, they would have you believe, is no longer aspirin. It's a whole new way of life.

Ben Gordon, the energetic staff economist for Senator Gaylord Nelson's Monopoly Subcommittee of the Select Committee on Small Business, has gathered together some illuminating advertisements and TV commercials of various analgesics that are so flagrantly idiotic that it is a wonder they sell any product. But they obviously do, or they wouldn't be continuing in such dismal proliferation.

One of them shows a woman sitting in a chair on her terrace, and the caption educates us to the questionable fact that Bayer works wonders when we're feeling so headachy, tense, and irritable that the simplest chore or disturbance becomes an irritation. But hold everything—Bayer Aspirin turns that mood around in a jiffy.

There is no medical substantiation that tension or irritation or mood changes can be relieved by aspirin, though it can bring relief from mild to moderate pain.

Another advertisement for Anacin would have you, the consumer, learn that this pill is less irritating, faster acting, and relieves tension. There is no evidence to support any of these claims. Further, the advertisement quite understandably fails to point out that Anacin quietly sneaked phenacetin out of its formula some time ago, when it was discovered that serious side effects, especially to the kidneys, resulted from its use. The manufacturer has never bothered to announce this change to the public.

An Excedrin ad that claims it has extra strength goes on to say: "Most headache tablets rely mainly on one ingredient, aspirin. Excedrin has four ingredients, including aspirin. Excedrin is an extra-strength pain reliever." The FDA's Dr. Henry Simmons commented on this: "We have no evidence as to the significance of the presence of four ingredients or the presence of an extra grain of aspirin." His latter words referred to a slight extra portion of aspirin in the pill, the effect of which would be totally unmeasurable by current study techniques.

One study did seem to give Excedrin a slight edge in relieving some pain, but in using this as a sales gimmick, Bristol-Myers, the makers, failed to point out that Excedrin is simply a bigger tablet than aspirin and that it produces more intestinal upset than two other brands of aspirin when used in equal tablet dose.

Bufferin is no less ridiculous in its advertising approach. A television commercial for the product advances this illuminating bit of information:

STUDENT: Why don't you listen to us? This college has got to change.
PROFESSOR: Agreed.
STUDENT: But not your way.
PROFESSOR: All right. Regrettably. Now can we keep our cool and all get together here at six?
STUDENT: O.K.
NARRATOR: Often people who are sensitive to others can be more sensitive to headache pain. Bufferin is for these people. Its strong medicine treats you gently. Plain aspirin is fine, but Bufferin goes to work much faster yet is actually gentler to your stomach. Because tough problems are tougher for sensitive people, we believe that strong medicine you need should treat you gently. Faster, gentler Bufferin. Strong medicine for sensitive people.

Dr. Elmer Gardner, a psychiatrist with the FDA, feels that this ad has implications far beyond the relief of pain and, thus, far beyond the claims that could legitimately be made by Bufferin. In other words, the ad was flatly misrepresenting the product. There is no evidence that Bufferin *is* gentler or faster acting.

A fascinating story of intramural contradiction arises from the advertising of three separate analgesic products put out by the same company, Sterling Drug.

One of Sterling's Bayer Aspirin ads asks: "Is there any way to improve on Bayer Aspirin to make it stronger? Well . . . suppose you buffered it, or combined it with other drugs, fizzed it, or tried to find a stronger ingredient and gave it a fancy name. First of all, aspirin is already the strongest pain reliever you can buy . . . buffering does not add speed or gentleness either. None is faster or more effective than Bayer Aspirin. Even we cannot improve it, although we keep trying."

Next, Sterling's own Vanquish ad says: "And Vanquish has a unique way of doing it—relieving headache—with extra strength and gentle buffers. Vanquish gives you extra strength and gentle buffers. It is the only leading pain-reliever you can buy that does."

On the heels of these two utterly contradicting ads by the same company, Sterling continues its capers with its ad on Cope:

"Think about the pain-reliever that you are using now. If it is one of the old established leading brands it cannot say what Cope says. More important, it cannot do what Cope does because Cope is different. . . ."

"The feeling I get from these three ads," says Dr. William Beaver, "is that somebody must be lying."

Not only was Sterling Drug contradicting itself on its three own products, but Cope has ingredients within it that contradict themselves. It has plain, old-fashioned aspirin. It has less, of course, than an ordinary aspirin tablet, because it has to make room for two other ingredients: methapyriline (an antihistamine) and caffeine. The antihistamine might possibly make you drowsy, but caffeine wakes you up. So the two ingredients are in there antagonizing each other. But beyond that, as Dr. Beaver notes, neither of them are in there in sufficient quantity to have any effect. The caffeine dose is about equal to that in a quarter of a cup of coffee.

Much has been said earlier about aspirin, its good qualities and dangers. But few people keep in mind that it is the leading cause of drug-induced, accidental, fatal poisoning in children, and this is worth repeating. For adults who have an allergy to it, it can be fatal. It frequently causes gastrointestinal bleeding, ulceration and, in rare cases, massive upper gastrointestinal hemorrhage. It is for this reason that it should be avoided when abdominal pain or an ulcer condition exists. It is particularly dangerous to those with bleeding disorders or who are taking anticoagulant or antidiabetic drugs. Nearly 70 percent of patients taking aspirin show a recurrent loss of blood of half to one full teaspoon of blood a day, and 10 percent of these lose two teaspoonfuls. No warning for any of these problems can be found on any aspirin label. People constantly ignore the commonsense rule to take a *full* glass of milk with aspirin or its compounds, along with a tablespoonful of an antacid like Maalox or, better yet, a good "house" brand generic antacid at often half the price. A little snack before taking aspirin wouldn't hurt either. Aspirin preparations that come out slightly more favorably as far as gastric side effects are concerned are the seltzer types, such as Alka-Seltzer, where both the water and the alkaline solution tend to help the aspirin to be absorbed more quickly.

If the television commercials would devote themselves to factual information, there might be some excuse for the millions of dollars spent on the atrocious chain of outright lies the commercials carry with them. The viewer can do nothing better than to recognize that there is little or no validity whatever to practically all the manufacturers' advertising claims.

The consumer must keep the essential truths about painkillers in mind in order not to be hoodwinked by this growing and deliberate hoax that the over-the-counter drug manufacturers are foisting on to the public.

There are only *three* effective pain-killers available over the counter, none of them being "mood" drugs. They are: aspirin, phenacetin, and acetaminophen. They are disguised in all kinds of combinations and trade names.

Nothing over the counter can surpass plain aspirin for pain relief, fever reduction, or cutting down inflammation in some conditions. Its scientific name is acetylsalicylic acid. All aspirin is made according to USP standards, and an unadvertised brand at 19 cents per hundred is just as safe and effective as Bayer Aspirin at 90 cents per hundred.

For those who can't tolerate aspirin, there is acetaminophen. It is about ten times as expensive, and it's just about as effective in killing pain and reducing fever. It is not as good as an anti-inflammatory agent.

Phenacetin is very poor in combating this latter condition, it is seldom used alone, and it has serious side effects if taken over a period of time.

"Extra strength" pain relievers such as Excedrin and Anacin are absurd promotional products, a glint in an advertising copywriter's eye, which have slightly more aspirin in them (not enough to make a discernible difference), cost more, and the other ingredients in them add little or nothing, except danger from side effects. As FDA's Dr. Henry Simmons said: "These and other analgesic products make promotional claims on all such preparations that have no real advantage over an equivalent dose of regular aspirin. There are many combination drugs that contain aspirin, phenacetin, or acetaminophen. The most widely known is APC, a combination of aspirin, phenacetin, and caffeine. Caffeine is present in an ineffective dose. Phenacetin involves potential hazards. And the entire preparation is no more effective for pain than aspirin."

When Bristol-Myers launched its highly doubtful product Excedrin P.M. on an unsuspecting public in recent years, it did so with considerable fanfare. Here was something new, we were led to believe, a "nighttime pain reliever" that, even though its $1.39 price for fifty tablets was twice the cost of plain, old, ordinary Excedrin, had a special formula that would take care of both pain and insomnia with one fell swoop. The "special formula" consisted of the same, tired ingredients as regular Excedrin, although Bristol-Myers yanked out the useless caffeine from that and threw in an antihistamine that may or may not make some people drowsy. Since a new drug has to be proved safe and effective for the FDA, it must go through the usual clearance. But Bristol-Myers, while trumpeting its "new" discovery to the public, refused to clear the drug with the FDA on the grounds that it wasn't a new drug at all, simply a combination of old ingredients. Federal marshals dispensed by the FDA whisked to a warehouse and seized forty cases of the product, and the legal fight is presently up for grabs. Meanwhile, Bristol-Myers continues to tout its tired product under a new name.

This sort of absurdity is happening constantly. A "pep" drug called Vivarin was advertised mawkishly, with a housewife describing how she was boring her husband to death, until she took a couple of Vivarin. Now he's sending flowers to her with a note reading: "To my new wife." The advertisement fails to mention that the product has little else in it beside caffeine, and that only equal to about half a cup of coffee per tablet.

About the only thing left to cheer about in the analgesic arena is that a pain reliever known as acetanilide has been disappearing from the combination products, although it used to be in a great many. You could easily spot a person who used this type of product regularly, because his entire body appeared to be covered with a blue-gray veil and his fingernails, nose, and lips took on a blue coloration.

In addition to the attention Senator Gaylord Nelson's subcommittee is turning to the inordinate promotion of over-the-counter drugs, Representative Paul Rogers of Florida, chairman of the House Subcommittee on Public Health, was not at all happy with the way the manufacturers were plugging their relax-and-pep-up pills on television. He feels, along with others, that such advertising could be a major contributor to the problems of drug abuse. He pointed his finger at Bristol-Myers, J. B. Williams, Whitehall Labs,

Block Drug, Miles Labs, and Jeffrey Martin Labs—makers respectively of NoDoz, Sominex, Sleep Eze, Nytol, Nervine, and Compoz. He extended his concern to the manufacturers of amphetamines and barbiturates, backing up a proposal that would put a lid on the number of these pills each manufacturer could turn out each year.

While this class of drug is supposed to be a prescription item—and it often is prescribed far too frequently—it more often than not turns up on the illegal under-the-counter market. Meanwhile, the big pharmaceutical houses pretend that they don't see how their products could *possibly* find their way into illegitimate channels. A local California assemblyman was so angered at Eli Lilly and Bates Laboratories because so many of their "speed" and barbiturate pills were finding their way into Mexican pharmacies and then into illegal channels, that he made both companies the target of a California Assembly resolution.

Since nearly 40 percent of the amphetamine pill production in the country cannot be accounted for, even by the Bureau of Narcotics and Dangerous Drugs, the situation shapes up almost as absurdly as the *New Yorker* cartoon about water pollution. The manufacturers' pronouncement with a straight face that there is no "recognition of the intensive efforts principal producers of amphetamines have made to curb illicit traffic" is one of the more incredible statements on the current drug scene. C. Joseph Stetler, president of the Pharmaceutical Manufacturers Association, said indignantly: "These companies maintain extraordinary precautions to prevent illegal diversion." It is hard to reconcile a leakage of nearly half of the total production in the country with this statement, and the PMA doesn't even match the politeness of the environmental polluter who said: "Gee, thanks for pointing that out."

Stetler was reacting to an FDA order announced by Commissioner Edwards to cut down the prescription use of amphetamine drugs sharply. The order limited their use to: uncontrollable sleepiness (narcolepsy), hyperkinetic disorders in children, and short-term treatment of obesity. This would make quite a dent in the 3.5 billion amphetamine dosage units that were made in this country during one recent year.

The whole scene concerning diet and reducing pills remains chaotic, as it has been over the past several years. The FDA will say with absolute certainty that there is no drug that will melt away fat. A restricted diet and exercise is the only thing that will work.

Some drugs can curb the appetite, but it is only safe to take them under the direction of a doctor.

After a big run on thyroid-amphetamine combination pills as an alleged treatment for obesity, a National Academy of Sciences panel determined that they were neither safe nor effective. The FDA requested manufacturers to remove them from the market, and after a long hassle, all but six agreed to do so. The last step in the drive was the recall of over 3,000,000 Obestat-Ty-Med tablets by the Lemmon Pharmacel Company, under FDA's prodding. The action was taken so vigorously after it became apparent that at least thirty-five people had died after taking the diet medication.

The ubiquitous J. B. Williams Company, along with its overenthusiastic advertising agency, Parkson, found itself faced with a cease-and-desist order from the FTC for its so-called 7-Day Reducing Program, consisting of wafers and alleged diet drink mix. The FTC charged that neither of these would cause the consumer to lose weight or inches, that similar types of diet plans were available at little or no cost, and that the protein product was of no significant value and unnecessary for weight reduction.

The boundary line between foods and over-the-counter drugs becomes thin when foods like this masquerade as drugs or dietary supplements. It can even happen to breads. ITT's Continental Baking Company has been a consistent and flagrant offender in misleading advertisements in the eyes of the FTC. For years, youngsters and mothers have been led to believe that Wonder Bread "helps build strong bodies 12 different ways." It took until 1971 for the FTC to order Continental Baking to stop any advertising of Wonder Bread unless 25 percent of the ad clearly and conspicuously disclosed that the FTC has alleged that Wonder Bread has been falsely advertised as more nutritious and appropriate for children than other enriched breads.

And the order goes further. Any future advertising must state in similar terms that Continental's Profile bread has been falsely advertised as effective for weight reduction. (Several breads, such as Hollywood Bread, are facing this charge, on the basis that the "diet" factor simply consists of slicing the bread thinner.)

The same company's Hostess Snack Cake faces the same fate. Its advertising must announce that these cakes have been falsely advertised as a major nutritional breakthrough, in the same manner as its fellow products above.

Beyond the analgesic, mood-booster, and diet rainbow, the rest of the over-the-counter drug picture is hardly more encouraging, especially in relation to wild, unsubstantiated claims that assault the airwaves and advertising pages daily. Many mystical nostrums survive under what is called a grandfather clause, somewhat of an equivalent to the GRAS list in food additives. In other words, if they don't kill you, and if you can still stand up after taking them, the FDA will allow you to buy them, and the rest is up to you and your conscience—to say nothing of the conscience of the company that is willing to take your money. If they show a real danger, the FDA can act, laboriously of course, through the long, tough litigation channels. The National Academy of Sciences has only been able to review 400 out of the more than 100,000 over-the-counter drugs. Since 85 percent of these have not shown adequate evidence to be considered "effective for their intended use," this could mean there are 85,000 different kinds of useless preparations on the market. The public is barely aware of which of these drugs are worthless, because the legal and public-notice measures the FDA must take are as sticky as treacle.

Just how Geritol has gotten away with its extravagant claims for over ten years is hard to explain. The Federal Trade Commission, which is responsible for keeping revved-up advertising agencies under control, is locked in combat with Geritol over the problem. FTC's gripe about the product is that its advertising is designed to make any consumer feel that Geritol will handily take care of tiredness, loss of strength, and any rundown feeling that many people complain of a considerable percentage of the time. Now the Geritol ads openly invite everyone to diagnose himself and come up with the inevitable conclusion that he has an iron deficiency.*

In the first place, this is not true. Iron deficiency is not this common. In the second place, iron fortification can be deadly if overdone, as recorded earlier in this book. In the third place, iron deficiency anemia is impossible for a person to diagnose by himself. To suggest such a possibility is to victimize people, as Dr. Robert Pitofsky, of the Federal Trade Commission, will tell you. The J. B. Williams Company, makers of Geritol, and its fellow agency, Parkson Advertising, are being sued by the FTC for $1,000,000 in civil penalties because the advertising that followed after an FTC order to cease and desist was as misleading as the former advertising. The advertisements continued to suggest that tiredness is inevitably linked with iron deficiency, yet they failed to disclose that the great majority of tired people have no iron deficiency problem.

The feeling of nausea created by a Geritol TV commercial could likely upset any possible benefit the nostrum might have. You might see a wife sitting on a chair, as if she's posing for a family portrait. Then you hear her say:

> I'm going to admit something that many women hesitate to admit. I'm a housewife and I'm proud of it. Sure I have to pick up after my children, walk the dog. But I love being a housewife and one of the reasons I'm able to is because I take good care of myself. I exercise, watch my diet, try to get enough rest and to be sure I get enough iron and vitamins, I start every day with a Geritol tablet. I do a lot for my family. Geritol is one of the nice things I do for myself.

* At one point, the FTC gave Geritol an ultimatum to get rid of the expression "iron power" from its advertising, but this was only one of many incidents over a decade of battles.

And then, persistently in practically all these commercials, the announcer's voice-over says: "Geritol every day."

This commercial appeared in 1971. Back in 1968, the FTC wrote in its decision:

> The commercials broadcast by Geritol since the order [of November 24, 1967] in this matter became final, not only fail to comply with the order but, in many instances, have so forcefully left the viewer with the overall impression—*i.e.*, that Geritol is a generally effective remedy for tiredness—that they are no less, objectionable than the commercials denounced by the Commission when it issued the original order.

The whole vitamin alphabet is being overpromoted, oversold, and overused. The final report of the panel concerned with this for the National Academy of Sciences drug study states quite bluntly:

> The panel does not recognize the need for multi-vitamin supplementation in healthy individuals who have an adequate diet. However, the panel does recognize the need for multiple-vitamin and mineral preparations in certain segments of the population. It also recognizes the lack of precise data on which rational formulation can be based.

The report then goes on to warn about preparations containing disproportionate amounts of potentially hazardous nutrients, both vitamins and minerals. Among the worst of these are vitamins A and D, fat soluble vitamins, plus, of course, the dangers of taking in too much iron.

The principal use for vitamin preparations, according to FDA specialists, is for infants, the young, and pregnant women. Since no individual can accurately diagnose the cause of persistent tiredness, overdoing vitamin intake can be dangerous. It is almost universally known that vitamins in the B-group and vitamin C are water soluble and therefore are not stored in the body. But since vitamins A, D, E, and K are fat soluble, they are stored and can be toxic. Vitamin manufacturers are specifically prohibited from claiming that vitamins and minerals can replace food, take the place of sleep or rest, ease tension, restore youth, grow hair, restore sexual powers, build muscles, curb appetites, or cure serious diseases, according to FDA guidelines.

The run on vitamin C as a cure and preventive for the common cold sprang from the views of Dr. Linus Pauling, a Nobel Prize winner in chemistry, whose ideas are certainly not to be tossed aside lightly. Drugstores have been hard put to keep vitamin C in stock. Since Dr. Pauling recommended as much as 15 grams of vitamin C a day after a cold sets in and 1 to 5 grams as a preventive, this is understandable.

The problem is that in spite of Dr. Pauling's eminence, his conclusions were based on very shaky and uncontrolled research studies. One of them involved only twenty-two subjects, among whom were several dropouts. Another involved an animal study, the main thrust of which was a subjective statement by the biochemist who conducted it on the state of his own well-being after taking 3 to 5 grams of vitamin C daily for a ten-year period. As the authoritative *Medical Letter* pointed out, "A controlled trial of the effectiveness of vitamin C against upper respiratory infections must be conducted over a long period and include many hundreds of persons to give meaningful results. No such trial has been performed."

Further, the *Medical Letter* went on to say that vitamin C in large doses *can* have adverse effects, stones in the urinary tract being among them. Very large doses of anything can be suspect. The publication concluded its comment on the subject by saying:

Professor Pauling himself says that "So far as I am aware, no large scale study, involving several hundred or thousand subjects, has been carried out to show to what extent the regular ingestion of ascorbic acid [vitamin C] in large amounts is effective in preventing and ameliorating the common cold and associated infections." In the light of this statement, it is difficult to understand his going to the public with recommendations that are bound to be widely accepted.

Later research studies agreed with the *Medical Letter*'s caution.

With regard to cough medicines, the same publication, which is considered one of the most objective and authoritative in the medical field, was not much more encouraging. It suggested that that miserable tickle in the throat can be handled just as handily with a candy drop as with potentially hazardous medication. The tendency of cough-mixture makers to load up a syrup or pill with four or more drugs at one time can multiply the chance for adverse reactions. Again, well-controlled tests are lacking, and the piling together of so many drugs in one bottle usually results in the patient getting less than enough of each of the individual ingredients, any one of which might be better than the weakened combination.

Further, coughing is a needed reflex action to get rid of secretions, and if it is suppressed too much, it can be harmful. The editors of the *Medical Letter* leaned toward the use of steam or cool mist rather than loading up with drugs. (Warnings are out on vaporizers, though. Many children have been severely scalded by them.) Since coughs are most frequently self-limiting and usually do not develop into serious illnesses, the less medicine, the better. The mixtures on the patent medicine market are loaded with multiple and sometimes conflicting drugs and therefore increase the possibility of adverse reactions.

The National Academy of Sciences drug review panel went along with this cautious approach. Since coughing is a nonspecific symptom that covers a multitude of possible illnesses, a genuinely persistent cough calls for a lot more attention than an over-the-counter medicated cocktail. The panel emphasized that the underlying cause of the cough is the most important thing to get at. The panel also agreed that coughs can play a protective role, can get rid of unwanted secretions and promote drainage. If an over-the-counter cough medicine masks symptoms, it is certainly doing more harm than good. The NAS panel suggested that if a temperature of over 100° sets in and lasts for more than three days, if there are chills and marked weakness, if there is chest pain, shortness of breath, wheezing, thick or colored sputum, or blood-streaked sputum, the only answer is an immediate trip to the doctor. Most of the decongestants or expectorants available over the counter are worth very little, especially in doses present in the bottles on the drugstore shelves.

Another property of cough medicines is their attraction as "kick-inducers." Some of them have as much as 50 percent alcohol, about equivalent to that of 100-proof whiskey. A pharmacist from Wisconsin told the story of a young married woman who made alarmingly frequent visits to his drugstore to buy Vicks Formula 44. Sometimes she bought as many as three bottles a day. She explained this all by saying that her children had chronic coughs, or that she was buying for a neighbor, or that she had dropped a bottle on the way home —a variety of excuses. When several other pharmacists reported the same problem, they finally agreed to tell her that there would be no more sales unless she brought a letter from her doctor. The end of the story is uncertain, because there was a plentiful supply on the open supermarket shelves, where she could continue to fulfill her uncontrolled yearnings.

People like this are called floaters by the pharmacists and obviously are in need of psychiatric help. Some will have an uncontrolled urge for a product like iron tablets, which are, of course, specifically for anemia and are extremely dangerous in excess and to children. Most druggists will spot this hazardous practice, but again the supermarket shelves will beckon and afford a peaceful anonymity for the unfortunate floater.

When Vicks brought out its cough mixture Nyquil, it was not only a temptation for the floater (25 percent alcohol), but the same history repeated itself as with Excedrin P.M. In its typical medicine-man drum beating, Vicks claimed the product as a brand-new breakthrough: "NEW" screamed their headline in a druggists' promotion piece. "Vicks Nyquil—the nighttime cold medicine that's going to make cold tablets move over!"

But was it new when the FDA reminded Vicks that as a

new drug, it had to be registered and proven safe and effective for its intended use? Not by a long shot. Vicks claimed that Nyquil was just made up of the same old ingredients that had been knocking around for a long time. So Nyquil rests on the market without a new drug approval and will fight any attempt by the FDA to brand it a new drug. To Vicks, it's nice to have it both ways.

A very neat promotional scheme was influential in making the public believe that Coricidin was an especially effective remedy for colds. Realizing that the recommendation of the pharmacist is a powerful sales influence, the Coricidin manufacturer cooked up a scheme whereby a "mystery shopper" would circulate among drugstores all over the country. He would enter the stores, posing as someone stricken with a cold, and ask the various druggists what they would recommend. If the man behind the counter recommended Coricidin, the "mystery shopper" would present him with a fat $50 check and move on to the next store. Very few of the public knew about this persuasive little scheme, which had nothing whatever to do with the value of the product as a medicine. It just seemed that way.

As a matter of fact, long and carefully controlled studies have shown that medicines that include antihistamine ingredients like Coricidin neither shorten the duration nor reduce the severity of the common cold, according to Dr. Philip Norman, of the Johns Hopkins School of Medicine. In addition, they have the serious side effects of producing drowsiness (practically all of the over-the-counter sleeping aids use them as their basic active ingredients). "The only possible value of antihistamines for cough lies in their sedative action," Dr. Norman stated, "and straight sedative drugs are as useful and probably more so." In certain allergies and in hay fever, the use of antihistamines under medical supervision is effective. Dr. Frances Lowell, chief of the allergy unit of the Massachusetts General Hospital, pointed this out but added: "I agree that all the evidence indicates that antihistaminic drugs are not effective in the common cold." Speaking specifically of Coricidin-D, Dr. Lowell stated: "The only possible use for this particular combination would be for the common cold, and I would not prescribe it for the common cold or anything else, for that matter."

Phenylephrine, another component of Coricidin, received short shrift from the *Medical Letter*, which said: "There is no acceptable evidence that vasopressor 'decongestant' drugs, such as phenylephrine, which are present in many cough mixtures, are useful in relieving coughs of any kind."

All of this turbulent, towering scene is in broad view of Washington officials, members of Congress, manufacturers, advertising agencies, and consumers—but it is still going on. If it is "totally out of control," as many thoughtful and responsible people think, what can be done about it? Senator Gaylord Nelson's and Congressman L. H. Fountain's subcommittees are the most active on the scene, but they cannot be expected to do the whole job of curbing this massive imposition on the public. Ralph Nader and his Center for the Study of Responsive Law are doing incredible work with a minuscule budget. The FDA and the FTC have got to be given credit for keeping a couple of thumbs in the dike, but except for a couple of minority members of the Federal Communications Commission, this agency's concern is shockingly indifferent to the very real dangers of the over-the-counter drug fest.

When FCC (Federal Communications Commission) Chairman Dean Burch stated publicly and with a straight face that TV advertising revenues for headache cures, sedatives, and stimulants was $111,000,000 in 1970 and added: "Neither benefits nor revenues should be undermined unless the case to do so is truly established," he was hardly giving a priority to consumer safety or to the consumer's financial protection from being bilked of his money on ineffective products.

One of Burch's own commissioners of the FCC, Nicholas Johnson, took an exactly opposite view. He felt that the advertising of "mood" drugs was much worse than the cigarette commercials used to be. Referring to Burch's surprising statement, Johnson said:

I regret to say that the response of the broadcasting industry to the mountains of evidence of its adverse impact is not encouraging. . . . Now you hear the same argument—only this time from the FCC—that we must not act too hastily to remove drug advertising from the airwaves because it produces over $100,-000,000 a year for the broadcasters!

Commissioner Johnson came out directly with the suggestion that all over-the-counter drug advertising should be banned outright or, at the least, cleared with both the FDA and the FTC before being aired. He concluded his statement to Senator Nelson's subcommittee by saying:

Ralph Nader has taught us many things. One of the most important is that we as human beings have a right to hold decision makers personally accountable for their acts—whether they participate in decisions in corporations or in government. They are people who are making the conscious decisions that harm peoples' lives, and fail to make the most of the opportunities they have to enrich the life of our nation. We ought to ask them personally how they can justify what they decide to do—whether it is a network president, a product manufacturer, an advertising agency executive, or a Federal Communications Commissioner.

16

A Second Brief Slice of Time

BY THE time 1972 came into being, the dreary news was continuing at the same pace as it had in the opening months of 1971. That sample slice of time, discussed in the opening chapter, was easily matched by the threats to consumer safety emerging during the waking hours of 1972. It is almost safe to predict that things will continue this way until the food, drug, and cosmetic industries are adequately controlled, instead of coddled, by friendly government agencies.

Bess Myerson Grant, the fiery Commissioner of Consumer Affairs for New York City, started the New Year off by telling a New York *Times* reporter: "It is time to stand up against the degradation of our food supply. Lobbyists and food-processing interests are manipulating Federal agencies to legitimize the adulteration of our food and drink." Among the manifold problems in this area, Mrs. Grant had singled out hot dogs and orange juice as choice examples. The popular American snack of a hot dog and orange drink might consist only of a melange of fat, corn syrup, and a batch of chemicals for the meat; water and chemicals with a splash of orange juice for the beverage. She branded the U.S. Department of Agriculture's new proposal to let the hot dog manufacturer throw in sodium acid pyrophosphate for "cosmetic" purposes to make the hot dog pink as "truly contempt for the consumer."

She pointed out that the so-called all-meat frankfurters are packed with some chemicals that have never been tested. In addition to beef and pork, a typical all-meat frankfurter includes corn syrup, dextrose, flavoring, erythorbic acid, sodium nitrate, sodium nitrite, salt, and water.

Cosmetics reentered the scene as 1972 gathered momentum. The President's National Commission on Product Safety issued a report that some 60,000 women each year suffer from skin eruptions, loss of hair, marked allergic reactions, burns, and itching—a category adding up to the second largest personal injury claims in the nation's insurance companies. But these were considered only a fraction of the injuries sustained. The cosmetic industry association was continuing its fight to keep the consumer buying blind, without the listing of ingredients on the labels and plugging for "self-regulation." By April, 1972, the FDA quietly bowed to industry pressure and bought the industry's "voluntary" plan. Such plans have consistently been worthless as far as consumer protection is concerned. About the only bright spot consisted of Avon Products' concession to send out a list of ingredients in its products on request.

A new and expanded thalidomide-type crisis may have been avoided in March, 1972, when an Australian gynecologist found that seven babies had been born without arms in the Sydney area, after some of their mothers had taken a tranquilizer known as imipramine during the early months of pregnancy. The drug is more widely known under its trade name, Tofranil. CIBA, the Swiss manufacturer, felt that it had done its duty in a label warning against the use of the drug for pregnant women—although this obviously had not worked in Australia.

The makers of ineffective vaccines were cited by Senator Ribicoff in a report released in the early spring of 1972. He struck out not only at the manufacturers, which included such companies as Eli Lilly, Merck, Sharp & Dohme, Merrell, Hoffman, and Parke-Davis, but also at the U.S. Division of Biological Standards, which failed to reject the vaccines. About the only thing that some of these diluted vaccines can create are side effects. One product alleged to be effective in the treatment of upper respiratory infections, bronchitis, infectious asthma, and other disabilities often caused fever, rash, abdominal cramps, and diarrhea in children. Another worthless vaccine for eye inflammation can create chills and fevers up to 104°, muscular pains, and malaise.

Aspirin continued to be in the news in 1972. A team of doctors at the University of Virginia Medical School felt that aspirin bottles should contain sharp warnings against the frequent adverse reactions it causes in damages to eyes, kidneys, and liver—to say nothing of the burns it can cause in the digestive tract. Nearly 5 percent of the cases studied by the medical team revealed adverse reactions from aspirin.

Serious questions about Dr. Linus Pauling's vitamin C regimen for preventing colds made the new year glum for those who were taking massive doses of the vitamin for this reason. A University of Maryland research team found "no preventive or therapeutic effectiveness of vitamin C against the common cold in the subjects studied with the dosage level used."

Recalls continued at their usual rate. Over 3,000,000 cans of Coca-Cola, Fanta, and Sprite were whisked off the market in New York State by the FDA, after many aluminum lids on the cans were discovered to be contaminated with a solvent.

The jolly ambiance of Christmas was threatened by the discovery that the sparkling foil icicles made to hang from Christmas trees contained up to 97.4 percent lead—which could be fatal to children if eaten. Manufacturers were said to have agreed with the FDA to take them off the market for 1972.

A more serious problem with lead came up with the discovery that Crest toothpaste tubes had a 99-percent lead content, according to the Scientists' Institute for Public Information—a sharp threat to children who might chew on them. *Environment* magazine indicated that a study showed that none of the other tubes tested had more than 0.2-percent lead in them.

Meanwhile, sinus sufferers were finding little comfort in

the fact that many drugs containing phenylpropanolamine hydrochloride (PPM) were exposing them to many side effects. These included tremor, weakness, irregular heartbeat, dizziness, anxiety, insomnia, headache, tension, and sweating. Drugs containing PPM include Sinubid, Sinutab, Allerest, Trimanic, Tussagesic, and other over-the-counter cold and sinus remedies. The FDA failed to supply Chairman Fountain's investigating committee with the reasons why these products should remain on the market.

Stilbestrol was still very much in the news as 1972 began. The FDA finally got around to warning doctors not to prescribe the synthetic hormone for pregnant women after one medical journal's report on sixty cases of a cancer found in the reproductive tract of daughters of women who had taken the drug during pregnancy. Fountain's subcommittee chided the FDA for delaying the warning against diethylstilbestrol (DES) in pregnancy from March until November. In a rare, if ineffectual, case of alertness, the Department of Agriculture went through the motions of making cattlemen push back the time period to seven days before slaughter in which DES could not be used, but Congress felt this was still inadequate.

The biggest news breaking in early 1972 by far was the long-delayed hexachlorophene story. Just why it took so long to emerge on the front pages will remain one of the mysteries of the day. Even Ralph Nader was slow in taking action. In April, 1971, the brass of Armour-Dial had descended on Commissioner Charles Edwards' office at the FDA. The straws in the wind were obvious at that time. Yet it took until January 6, 1972, for the FDA to come out with an announcement that restrictions would be imposed on the use of the chemical. At this time, the FDA stated that "recent studies had raised questions about the use of hexachlorophene." No mention was made of the series of medical reports over the previous decade that had made it obvious that hexachlorophene was not to be toyed with. Even dermatologists seemed to be surprised by the new restrictions, many having habitually prescribed pHisoHex for the acne of teen-agers and for bathing babies and other vulnerable patients.

With the announcement came the inevitable howls from industry, not only from Sterling-Winthrop, which was facing the loss of a $15,000,000-a-year business in pHisoHex, but most particularly from the feminine spray manufacturers. Alberto-Culver's president, Leonard H. Lavin, blasted the ruling as the result of "negative-minded consumerist groups who would subject our entire economy to a Marxist purge of everything they object to." Even though many doctors had indicated that soap and water were far preferable for the service that the feminine sprays were supposed to perform, Alberto-Culver insisted that warnings about the use of the sprays were unnecessary. The company even demanded the dismissal of John Walden, the FDA public relations officer, an act approaching the sending of an affectionate cocker spaniel to the dog pound.

On the heels of the clampdown on pHisoHex came news that Yale University's nurseries, connected with the Yale Hospital, reported a sharp upturn in the presence of staph bacteria after the use of hexachlorophene soap had been curtailed. But not noticed by the general public was that it was at Yale that the first use of the hexachlorophene soap was branded as being effective against staph. This proprietary interest would have to be weighed very carefully against the precipitous haste with which the news from Yale was announced.

Further, by March, 1972, a series of tests at the Albert Einstein College of Medicine showed that hexachlorophene very definitely interfered with the ability of brain cells to produce the energy they need to function properly.

Counteracting the Yale story was an FDA official bulletin which read:

> Recent studies challenge the safety of hexachlorophene bathing of infants, a practice which has been widely advocated as effective prophylaxis against nursery epidemics of staphylococcal skin infections. A critical review of the studies on which this

claim is based indicates that whereas there is no doubt that hexachlorophene bathing decreases skin colonization of gram-posi-
tive organisms, there is a lack of substantial evidence that hexachlorophene washings by themselves prevent staphylococcal
disease or show antibacterial activity against gram-negative organisms. Hospitals are known to operate nurseries safely without
the use of this product.

A poignant case was revealed by *Medical World News* while
the FDA was making up its mind about releasing the re-
straining order on hexachlorophene. One woman who had
been using a vaginal spray with hexachlorophene was quoted
by the publication as saying: "It was the severest pain I've
ever had in my life. Childbirth was nothing compared to it."

Even the FDA had admitted that hexachlorophene is all
but useless in combating vaginal odor.

Feeble action at last came about in combating the over-
production of amphetamines, or "speed." But the action
again was accompanied by the howls of the drug manufacturers who had been turning out massive carloads of the
drug, much of which were often shipped to Mexico and then
back over the border to this country via illegal channels.
Ironically, a written recommendation to curb the production
was lost for two months in Washington's bureaucratic jungle.
Health authorities have long recognized that the overpro-
duction of amphetamines by "legitimate" drug manufacturers, and the freewheeling prescribing of the drug by some
doctors, had practically created an amphetamine epidemic.

The Bureau of Narcotics and Dangerous Drugs finally got
around to slashing the quota for manufacturers to about 70
percent of what the manufacturers wanted. Just why the
drug producers *wanted* to create so many pills is a little hard
to understand. The drug has only two legitimate uses: for the
narcolepsy patients, who can't keep awake; and for those
suffering from hyperkinesis, those with increased and uncontrollable muscular movements. About 600,000 cases in the
country would respond to treatment. A New York medical
group estimates that 1,200 kilograms of amphetamines would

take care of this need. Industry asked for nearly 20,000 kilograms, with no explanation as to where the balance of pills would be channeled. The FDA recommended a total production of about 8,500 kilograms, also with no explanation of where the excess pills might end up, especially since the use of amphetamines in weight reduction has been scorned by the medical profession. What it all adds up to is that the quota restrictions are most generous, being about seven times higher than needed. One company, a Penwalt Corporation subsidiary, had shipped to Mexico enough "speed" over a recent eighteen-month period to fill 45,000,000 capsules. Estimates are that about 60 to 70 percent of this is either smuggled back into the United States or sold without prescription in Mexico near the Texas border in *farmacias* standing in open fields.

At long last, the FDA review of over-the-counter drugs got underway at the beginning of 1972, with 100,000 nostrums up for review in a three-year study. Cold preparations, pain killers, mood drugs, stimulants, sedatives, and sleep aids will be the targets for this long-delayed project.

First on the list will be the antacids, which are supposed to neutralize acidity in the stomach. These have never stood high in the opinion of medical men. The over-the-counter pitchmen on radio and television will probably not enjoy the prospect of the review, but the consumers cannot help but benfit. Just how much money has been thrown down the drain on ineffective or even dangerous over-the-counter preparations cannot be estimated.

Meanwhile, 1972 didn't seem to offer too much hope in food protection. To cover some 500 food production plants, Connecticut had four FDA inspectors. In New York State, sixty-four FDA men were entrusted to the job of covering some 5,000 plants. In New Jersey, there were thirty inspectors to cover over 2,000 plants. The veil of protection remains thin.

By February, Senator Gaylord Nelson and his staff assistant, Judyth Robinson, ably shaped up and completed the Food Protection Act of 1972, which was presented to the

Senate as a Valentine's Day gift. The bill struck at the very critical weakness in present FDA procedures, whereby the manufacturer supplies his own tests on the safety and effectiveness of food additives. The objective of the legislation is to eliminate the use of unsafe, untested, and unnecessary chemicals in the food supply. It was just about a year before this that food and chemical industry spokesmen had made their classic statement that the industry had the right to make its own decisions on the status of what chemicals went into food, whether the FDA had approved them or not.

Said Senator Nelson: "I believe that it is time to find out which of the chemicals we are ingesting daily are safe from toxicity and long-range harmful effects, and how they react with other chemicals affecting the human body."

Certainly the mass of consumers would say "amen" to that. But for the food industry and their lobbyists, the inevitable counterattack would begin.

17

Rx for Action

THERE is plenty wrong, but there are certain things that can be done. Most important for the consumer is to be aware of what has happened, is happening, and will continue to happen without the counterforce of a vigorous consumer movement for safety, not just price protection. Price rigging is bad enough; the lack of safety is intolerable. Sometimes both are involved, as in prescription drugs where a captive audience must pay outrageous prices, dictated by the pharmaceutical cartel that is the equivalent of a monopoly, in order to stay alive. For the consumer to be aware, he must know and feel what is going on in those vital areas where he should be protected but isn't. Only then can he know what to fight and how to fight it.

Corporation venality is not just an acrimonious phrase or an empty incantation. It is real, vivid, and commonplace, as documented in the pages of this book and in scores of other places. To understand it is to know what must be overcome in the first line of self-protection. The most difficult—and most disillusioning—thing to realize is that corporation morality—or lack of it, rather—does not stem from a group of deliberately evil men who sit down to gamble with the consumer's life. What happens is that the individual in the corporation is caught up in a tidal force of which he is only a part, usually masked in anonymity and unable to do anything about it actively without being sacked.

Take the case of a former Merck, Sharp & Dohme executive whom we will call Charles Syndrome. Despite his ficti-
tious name, his is a very real, detailed case. As a leading promotion executive, he found himself under the usual pressure
of building up sales volume as high as it could be pushed.
This was, of course, the function of his job, and he accepted
the challenge. His associates were congenial, and as he observed later, they were men of basic goodwill who had families to support and made reasonably good salaries.

It wasn't long before he found that his sense of social responsibility became completely subordinated to the push for
profits. The strange part was that the large profits of the
company made very little difference to him personally.
Whatever bonus he would get would not be enough to be a
strong personal motivating force. As a game, he got caught
up in the corporate state and found himself riding along with
it.

One day near the end of a fiscal year, Merck found itself in
the position of simply making too much money. After the
long Kefauver hearings investigating the extravagant profits
of the ethical drug companies, this was a very sensitive
point. The reaction among the top brass at Merck was immediate. Charles was called to the office of a vice-president,
who laid the figures out on his desk and said: "What in the
hell are we going to do? We're making too much money. I
want you to get the promotion department off its tail and
figure out how we can get rid of all this excess money—fast."

Caught up with the urgency and the challenge, Charles
went back to promotion and started to work. Under his guid-
ance, elaborate promotion pieces to the doctors were planned
and rendered. Lavish brochures in four-color process plates
beautifully bound in buckram were planned. Even with a
large print order, the direct cost ran to 70 cents a copy. Post-
age to send them to the doctors came to 64 cents each.

While this was being done, a series of utterly useless high-
budget films were put into production. Grants were set up for
cooperative doctors, with the unspoken proviso, of course,

that they would use Merck drugs for their research and tests. In this practice, some would always report honestly and objectively, some would not. Advertising schedules in the medical journals were automatically doubled—a windfall to the publishers.

Meantime, the sick, the elderly, the young, and the dying were paying for this ultraplush promotion through rigged prices and many artificial patents that were meaningless as far as the patient was concerned. This bothered Charles, as did the rest of the gymnastics he found himself going along with.

"Merck, Sharp and Dohme spends a helluva lot on research," he observed later. "But most of it is pointed in one direction—to the drugs they can patent and clean up on. Exclusive properties. At one time they were spending around forty million dollars on research. Part of this was true and valid. But most of it was simply manipulating molecules, either to get around someone else's patent, or thinking up new combinations of old drugs to pack into one pill. These combination products would be absolutely useless, if not harmful, to the patient and cost him more money, to boot."

After a while, the situation began to get under Charles' skin. It became more and more obvious to him that the patient was in no position to question the kind of drug that was being prescribed for him and that the doctor, as the purchasing agent for the patient, was practically dependent on the drug company's detail man for his information. There was also the book called *The Physician's Desk Reference*. This, Charles felt, was a laugh because all it consisted of was a collection of information that the companies prepare about their own drugs. There are no purely generic drugs listed in it, so that the doctor has to look drugs up under their trade names. The publishers charge the drug companies to list their drugs, then give the books away free to physicians.

His disillusionment grew stronger by the day. He watched the Pharmaceutical Manufacturers Association fight against any legislation that would protect the consumer, the blindness of his peers and superiors to social needs, and the downright Machiavellian maneuvers the drug companies utilized to rig prices and promote useless nostrums.

Shortly before he quit, he noticed an advertisement in the leading medical journals for the "new" Warner-Chilcott (a division of Warner-Lambert) drug called Peritrate. The ad consisted of eight solid consecutive pages. The drug was an old turkey, discovered by the Swedes many years ago, and was supposed to be a long-acting blood vessel dilator, possibly for use in angina pectoris.

"I knew that Warner-Chilcott had spent little or nothing in research money to resurrect this oldie, and right at the start of the copy, they began stretching claims. The ad was a whopper—sea gulls against the sun, and all that sort of thing. The first thing I said to myself was: 'What am I doing in this business?' The second thing I said to myself was: 'This is sure as hell going to get Warner-Chilcott into trouble.' "

It did—but hardly enough. U.S. marshals seized a shipment of Peritrate, and Warner-Chilcott suffered the extreme pain of paying the court costs of $35 and marshals' fees of $25.88. Meanwhile, the sick and the elderly paid out over $18,000,000 for Peritrate* in 1966, quite a tribute to Warner-Chilcott's raw medicine-man huckstering.

If Charles Syndrome, who finally left Merck, Sharp & Dohme, can reflect the atmosphere of what is going on in the "ethical" drug business, Dr. Richard Burack can demonstrate one doctor's fight against inexorable forces of the industry. He is author of the book *The New Handbook of Prescription Drugs* and clinical associate in medicine and affiliate in pharmacology of the Harvard Medical School. For many years, he has been a respected member of the Harvard Medical Services of the Boston City Hospital, chairman of the Committee of Drugs and Medications of the New England Deaconess Hospital, and in January, 1971, he was named by

* Said the 1970 Warner-Lambert annual report: "Peritrate, the company's leading cardio-vascular drug, continued to be highly regarded by physicians for their treatment of angina patients during the past year." But the Federal Supply Agency made public in January, 1971, that Peritrate was to be removed from all government hospital formularies because it has never been shown to be effective by careful scientific tests.

Governor Francis Sargent as chairman of the newly formed Massachusetts Drug Formulary Commission.

He saw the advertising for Peritrate, too, the same eight-page spread with the beautiful sea gulls. In his book, he points out that Peritrate was simply a new name for what had been known generically as pentaerythritol tetranitrate and which had fallen out of favor and was hardly used at all until Warner-Chilcott dubbed it by its new name and promoted it extensively.

"This is a perfect example," Dr. Burack said, "of how, through massive promotion, a drug that is of questionable efficacy and is possibly even harmful, can be made popular. And how by fiddling with the dosage form, and adding some phenobarbital, the price can be exploded to yield a windfall of profit."

Speaking of Warner-Chilcott's exaggerated claims for the drug, he continued:

> They have attempted to make doctors believe that its use would diminish the likelihood of patients having major heart attacks, and have spent vast sums to that end on advertisements in major medical journals. The FDA charged that a mailing of the company was "false and misleading" since it was "contrary to fact," and the physician whose single, company-sponsored study formed the major basis for the claims dissociated himself from the ads for the drug and called them "distasteful."

The former chairman of Warner-Lambert, incidentally, is Elmer Bobst, who has taken a fatherly interest in Richard Nixon for many years. Bobst brought Nixon into Warner-Lambert's law firm, so that it became the firm of Nixon, Mudge, Rose, Guthrie, and Alexander. John Mitchell, later to become Attorney General, joined the firm and had his name popped on the shingle. When Nixon and Mitchell went to Washington, they kept in close touch with their old friend Elmer Bobst, the Warner-Lambert czar who was also known as the Vitamin King.

It is ironic that in August, 1970, Warner-Lambert, with its

questionable track record, decided to buy Parke, Davis, with its equally unpalatable history. Here is a potential of creating an amoral giant that would compound by logarithms its capacity for bilking the consumer. The original Warner company had been on the prowl for years, swallowing smaller companies whole. It began by taking over the Hudnut cosmetic line, moved along by picking up the Lambert Company, with its almost useless but profitable Listerine product, and then added the companies producing Bromo Seltzer, Smith Brothers Cough Drops, Sloan's Liniment, and others.

This concentration of power created by the new merger not only lessens competition in the already concentrated drug industry but combines two giants whose lack of corporate morals have been well documented.

The FTC in fighting the merger naturally received little support from John Mitchell's Department of Justice, and the case has dangled in uncertainty for considerable time. Mitchell made the pretense of disqualifying himself from the case because of his former association with Warner-Lambert's law firm, turning it over to one of his assistants. Just how an assistant, working in the shadow of his boss, would react to this sort of situation presents an interesting picture. It all adds up to a graphic illustration of what the consumer faces in trying to find protection from corporate venality on the one hand and friendly-to-industry government forces on the other. Both add up to the continuation of large-scale profit-taking as a priority over consumer protection.

Dr. Burack, who is one of the very few doctors in the country recognized as an authority in both pharmacology and internal medicine, blamed the 1,500,000 persons sent scurrying to the hospital each year because of drug side effects on the profit-taking of the drug companies. "A couple of dozen giant pharmaceutical houses have all but wrested from the medical leadership responsibility for the continuing education of the busy doctor in drug prescribing," he said. "It cannot be denied that the pharmaceutical industry exerts undue influence on the profession at every level, from the student to the busy practitioner to the professor and educator. Its tools are simple: money and flattery."

In his office, Dr. Burack has a shelf holding a small array of plastic bottles of generic drugs—those not marketed under a trade name. "These bottles," Dr. Burack explained, "hold just about all the drugs needed to treat 99 percent of the patients who come to a doctor. None of them are brand names, which means that a patient can get them for a fraction of the cost. But at the same time, he doesn't sacrifice quality, because USP or National Formulary standards must be followed by any manufacturer of an important drug."

Quoting John Adriani, chairman of the Council on Drugs for the American Medical Association, Dr. Burack said: "The question is not *should* we abolish brand names and use generic names, but *when?*"

Then Dr. Burack added: "I think it's obvious that the top echelons of the FDA are controlled by the pharmaceutical companies, and I think this makes it hell on the patient, who is the captive customer."

In spite of all this, it is important for the consumer to realize that the FDA Commissioner is not wholly to blame. He sits on an extremely warm chair. One FDA career executive put it this way: "Anybody who heads up the Food and Drug Administration has got himself automatically in a coronary vise. He's looking down the barrel of a lot of shotguns."

While the top FDA executives seem more inclined to favor industry and to be watchdogs with very soft barks, many others in the FDA down the line go along with the more prevalent feeling that industry has demonstrated beyond doubt that it cannot and will not regulate itself. "Left alone, all manufacturers are crooks," one FDA section head said bluntly. "They have one idea in mind that comes out in every case we prosecute: Who can corner the biggest market and make the biggest profit?"

Other FDA people on the action line are concerned about a variety of things that in turn affect the consumer seriously. New styles of hospital supplies, for instance, are being introduced so fast that it's almost impossible to keep up with them. They also escape the preclearance requirements of food additives and drugs. They include such things as disposable needles for injections, plastic containers for blood, and operating-room kits. Some are being made by companies who have had little or no experience in the drug field. All of those items such as therapeutic devices and cosmetics, with their legal loopholes, are of serious concern to the understaffed FDA personnel. "There are fearsome gaps in all the laws," said one FDA executive. "The axiom that nobody takes any action until a major tragedy occurs stands up 90 percent of the time."

As if the ordinary, everyday problems were not enough, FDA inspectors sometimes lead precarious lives. Their decisions can mean thousands, sometimes millions of dollars to a manufacturer. The inspector is overworked and very vulnerable. A lot is at stake. One inspector found himself closing in on a very serious health violation on the part of a small drug manufacturer suspected of illegal drug traffic. It became apparent that hundreds and thousands of dollars were involved, and the manufacturer did not like the outlook at all. Documenting the case took many months. As the inspector neared the end of his documentation, it became apparent both to him and the manufacturer that criminal prosecution would be inevitable.

But the manufacturer had not been idle during this time. He had opened a savings account *for* the inspector, *without* the inspector's knowledge, and had been regularly depositing several hundred dollars a month in it. By the time the case reached a crisis, the inspector received through the mail a neatly recorded savings bank book totaling over $10,000.

This was far from the old-fashioned bribe technique. This was blackmail. If the inspector brought the case to trial, the manufacturer would simply produce the evidence: a Xerox copy of the bank book to show that the inspector had been accepting regular monthly payoffs. Even though he knew nothing about this, how could the inspector prove otherwise?

The inspector did the only thing he could do: He tore up the bank book and went on with the case, which he won.

There is a general feeling among the FDA middle rankers that they are overworked and that the agency's budget is shortchanged by Congress. One pointed out that Congress literally appropriates more for the care and feeding of birds than it does for the FDA.

General chatter on Capitol Hill regarding the FDA is variable, depending on the point of view. Bob Bird, the former hard-hitting, free-swinging staff man for Senator Ribicoff, is a tough and intelligent consumer advocate who doesn't like to mince words.

"The problem with the FDA is this," he said. "The National Institute of Health looks down from its ivory tower on the FDA as cops. The FDA guys get desks. The NIH guys get plush labs. But what has happened is that toxicology is no longer just mouse-painting or rat-killing. The FDA guys resent the NIH attitude, and you can't blame them."

With a morale factor like this, the consumer suffers. And he suffers more when much of the critical testing and appraisal of food and drug products are shunted out of the FDA and into the National Academy of Sciences panels, which are often dominated by industry men. As Bob Bird put it: "Right now, the National Academy of Sciences is being constantly called on by the FDA to get them off the hook. The question comes up as to whether the NAS has now become the full deciding arm of the Food and Drug Administration. The industry men on the panels or those who are under obligation to industry create a situation which is like an author reviewing his own book."

This is not a healthy thing for the consumer. One NAS panel head has admitted to being on the payroll of three giant drug corporations: Smith Kline & French, Burroughs Wellcome, and Merck, Sharpe & Dohme. This is a financial conflict of interest he never saw fit to divulge to the FDA. He lent himself to signing a virulent and almost totally misleading letter against generic drugs at the request of the Pharmaceutical Manufacturers Association's chief executive officer, C. Joseph Stetler.

The PMA is one of the strongest lobbyists in the country, but there are plenty more to go around among those set up to resist consumer demands.

Peter Barash, a top staff aide for Congressman L. H. Fountain's hard-hitting Intergovernmental Relations Subcommittee, has his own very clear ideas about the lobbyists and President Nixon's real attitude toward consumer protection, as opposed to the words the President uses.

"There is no question that Nixon is in the pocket of the big business community. Consumerism puts him in a tough position. But the actions he takes, rather than his words, are obvious. For instance, he wouldn't even *receive* a Product Safety Committee Report."

The mystique of lobbying is always hard to figure out. A lobbyist is the salesman for a cause and, by definition, a nagging nuisance most of the time. How, then, do they get anywhere? They go and see members of Congress in their offices, but that can be a very unpopular pastime to a busy Congressman. They throw lavish parties, but that can be a pretty obvious ploy. They also arrange for, create, develop, and gather enormous campaign contributions—and there's the rub. Congressman Florence Dwyer, of New Jersey, lost thousands and thousands of dollars in campaign funds because of her firm defense of the consumer's interests. Other members of both Houses have suffered the same fate.

The irony of this lobbying lies in the gruesome fact that business groups can deduct lobbying costs and have been able to do so since 1962. But *consumer groups cannot.* Not only that, but these groups are not as informed and organized as the trade associations or the archaic U.S. Chamber of Commerce, and the only main tool they have is their conviction that they are on the side of the angels, as naïve as that sounds.

All of this boils down to three very specific things that the consumer must recognize:

1. Government regulatory agencies have major problems. They include lack of realistic budgets and a soft stand on industry among the top echelons. They cannot fully protect the consumer.
2. Industry greed and venality are documented, established, and a consistent way of life. Industry can never be self-regulated.
3. There are legal loopholes that are creating serious time bombs.

The proposal by the White House in July, 1971, to create a new Consumer Safety Administration built on but replacing the FDA is merely an organizational restructuring that will affect the consumer's problems very little. While it may have some administrative advantages, it doesn't deal with the gut issues above, which remain the same.

The Congressional proposal, announced in June, 1972, for an independent agency to replace the FDA is a healthier idea and should be pushed and supported by all consumer advocates.

To deal with the issues, the consumer has to assume something which is a little hard to do in this era, and that is that in the long run, democracy does make sense. Democracy doesn't need defense half as much as it needs rendition. This is, of course, easier said than done, and hardly anyone is naïve enough to think that the abuses of the democratic process don't often overwhelm its potential. For instance, industry is constantly expounding on the virtues of the free enterprise profit system, while it creates anything but free enterprise. It builds up profits for distribution to a meaningless minority of the population.

In all the major industries, free enterprise is a farce. With the large conglomerates gulping up the small to the point of economic indigestion, huge islands of "private" socialism are formed, some with budgets larger than most of our states. These "private" socialist islands join with others to freeze out competition, rig prices, and bilk the consumer. At the same time, over 90 percent of the employees work on job-evaluated incomes that are nothing more than civil service classifications. Rank-and-file employees rarely personally experience the incentives that a genuine profit system brings with it. If less than 10 percent of the population experiences profit incentives emotionally, how can it be claimed that a profit system realistically exists? If it did, the venality of the food and drug corporations would no longer be venality, because most of the consumers would be sharing whatever surplus their excess energies produced.

Since the consumer is dealing with private socialism, he must recognize this and try to make what is left of the democratic process work. His best place for a fighting chance is Congress, because Congressmen need votes, even in the face of huge lobbyist donations to their campaigns. The fact is that Congressmen *do* listen and *are* sensitive to the demands of their constituents, even if the motivation rests on sheer opportunism. Some of the more dedicated confreres are willing to stick their necks out for the sake of their constituents and let the lobbyists fall where they may.

You don't need to be a naïve admirer of democracy to sense the pulse of it around the House and Senate Office buildings. There *is* a responsiveness to the new wave of consumer indignation. One Senatorial aide said: "Letters keep pouring in, and a lot of it is the result of Ralph Nader's work. He gets the public mad. More people are taking action than ever before. We get more letters demanding safety in consumer products from people who invariably start a letter by saying, 'I've never written a letter like this before.' The theme is heavier in the want of protection against hazards than it is against prices—but the latter is important to them, too. And the big companies are aware of this new wave. They don't like it."

Congress is the best target for the concerned consumer and about the last outpost against the supercharged corporation lobbies, the weak-kneed attitude in the regulatory agencies, and an industry-oriented administration.

Specifically, there are five things to stress in writing Congressmen:

1. Urge them to provide the FDA with more funds so that it can operate realistically.
2. Urge them not to give in to industry pressure, because it is the consumer who elects them and not industry.
3. Urge them to continue investigative hearings into the food, drug, and cosmetic industries without letup. Urge them further to carry on watchdog hearings on all the regulatory agencies to avoid complacency. These include the Food and Drug Administration, the Federal Trade Commission, the Department of Commerce, and the U.S. Department of Agriculture, especially.
4. Urge them to resist administration pressure favoring industry over the consumer.
5. Urge them to continue to close the legal loopholes that permit cosmetics, therapeutic devices, and hazardous products to come on the market without prior safety testing. All such products should face the same requirements that drugs or food additives face.

Every letter that comes into a Congressman's office is read. The loss of a voter is a real and precarious thing for him.

Writing Congressmen may seem like a relatively mild antidote to the excesses of industry and the laxity of the regulating agencies, and it is. But since it is the only area where resistance can be developed, the greater the number of letters, the better the chance of strengthening that resistance.

Ralph Nader's Center for the Study of Responsive Law finds it most effective to operate through Congressional committees, as well as through the consumer groups such as the National Consumer League of Washington, which does the same thing. The Congressional committees which are dedicated to consumer protection are headed up by conscientious and able men who keep both the federal agencies and industry on their toes. Most effective are those headed by Senators Gaylord Nelson (Monopoly Subcommittee of the Select Committee on Small Business), Frank E. Moss and Philip A. Hart (Consumer Subcommittee of the Committee on Commerce), Abraham Ribicoff (Subcommittee on Executive Reorganization and Government Research of the Committee

on Government Operations) and by Congressman L. H.
Fountain (Intergovernmental Relations Subcommittee of the
Committee on Government Operations). Moral support of
their activities by letter can help keep continued watchdog
surveillance of both industry and indifferent government
agency attitudes.

The very fact that industry hates and fears these committees is ample evidence that they are doing an effective job.
For example, the trade publication *Drugs and Cosmetics Industry* published an editorial that read:

> Utilizing superb craftsmanship in the sophisticated use of
> communications, and constantly shifting targets when one be-
> comes either riddled or unproductive of headlines, the forces of
> consumerism of late have been riding high. The Ralph Naders,
> the Bess Myersons, the Gaylord Nelsons all give ample evidence
> that they well know how to make hay while the sun shines.

The point that the editorial avoids is: Why *shouldn't* consumers and consumer advocates use every legitimate tool at
their command to combat the abuses the entire population is
subjected to by the food, drug, and cosmetic industries?

The same advice given by the authors of *100,000,000 Guinea
Pigs* in 1933 unfortunately holds true just as much today as it
did when it was written some forty years ago. The writers
concluded:

> We suggest that in general you set yourself the task of making
> it less and less comfortable for your state and local health and
> food officials. Give your congressmen and senators, and your
> state legislators no rest until they sit in judgment on the work of
> the national food and drug administration and the local health
> and food control authorities.
>
> Above all, let your voice be heard loudly and often, in protest
> against the indifference, ignorance, and avarice responsible for
> the uncontrolled adulteration and misrepresentation of foods,
> drugs, and cosmetics. In this adulteration and misrepresentation
> lurks a menace to your health that ought no longer be tolerated.

Simply, what it all adds up to is the need for tougher laws and tougher enforcement of them. Or, to imitate the elegant simplicity of Albert Einstein, who reduced the entire universe to a simple formula: $S = TL + TE$.

S is for Safety. TL is for Tougher Laws. TE is for Tougher Enforcement. You—the voter and consumer—need only that simple formula to work as concerned citizens toward the common objective.

Index

Cancer-producing additives, and De-laney Amendment, 169–70, 176, 179–80, 181, 185. *See also* Car-cinogenicity
Canned foods, and food poisoning, 192–93, 199
Carbon tetrachloride
fire extinguishers, 223–24
poisoning, 222–25
Carcinogenicity, 26. *See also* Food ad-ditives
of cosmetics, 248
and food additives, 18, 35
Carmine, in eye shadow, 250
Carnation Instant Breakfast, nutritional claims of, 39
Carroll, F. E., 264
Carson, Jordan, 89
Carter Products, 101
Carter-Wallace, 101 n., 245
Cascade (detergent), 243
C. botulinum, 189–91. *See also* Bot-ulism
Center for Disease Control (Atlanta), 54, 55, 56
Center for the Study of Responsible Law, Ralph Nader's, 37, 172, 175, 283, 305. *See also* Nader, Ralph; Turner, Jim
Cēpacol Mouthwash and Gargle, 30, 252
Chadduck, H. W., 132
Charcoal briquettes, 243
Charles Pfizer and Co. Inc., 103, 117
and Drug Efficacy Study, 136
and Unburn, 255
Cheer (detergent), 243
Chemical Feast, The (Turner), 37, 171
Chemicals. *See also* Food additives, GRAS list
in foods, and GRAS review, 166–87
synthetic
accidental, 179
intentional, 179
Chemical Specialties Manufacturers Association, 232
Chemical Week, 255
Chemway Corporation, 253–54
Chicago, University of, 99
Child Protection and Toy Safety Act, 31
Children
aspirin poisoning in, 271
and bubble bath, dangers of, 256
and Chloromycetin, 68
drugs for, and drug labeling, 38, 100
and household hazards and danger-ous toys, 233–45
and household poisonings, 229–33
hyperactive, 100
as therapeutic orphans, 38
Children's Cancer Research Founda-tions, 179
Chloral hydrate, as effective sleeping pill, 108, 109
Chlor-alkali plants, mercury poisoning and, 204, 205, 206
Chloramphenicol (Chloromycetin), 38. *See also* Chloromycetin
Chlordane, 30

Chloromycetin (chloramphenicol), FDA investigation of, 64–78, 91
Chlorpromazine, 38, 101, 107
Choate, Robert, 34, 43
CIBA Pharmaceuticals, 30, 101, 136, 286
Citrus red 2, food coloring, 35
Clairol Silk and Silver, 246
Clams, and *Gonyaulax cantenella* con-tamination, 18
Clostridium perfringens, and food con-tamination, 197, 199
Coal-tar dyes, 184
use of, in cosmetics, 247–48
Coca-Cola recall, 287
Cochran, Samuel, Jr., 188–89
Cochran, Mrs. Samuel, 188–91
Codeine, 38, 109, 110
Code of Federal Regulations, 59
Cold Power (detergent), 243
Cold remedies, 282–83
Colgate Palmolive Company, 136
Chlorophyll Toothpaste with Gardol, 253
Dental Cream, 30, 253
Colmore, Dr. Henry, 188–89
Color Additive Amendments (1960), 184
Color additives, 35. *See also* Food additives
in cosmetics, 249–50
in food, 18, 178, 183–84
Combination drugs
antibiotic, 91–92
ban on, 138, 139
fixed, 141
Commoner, Barry, 24
Communicable Disease Center (At-lanta), 258, 259
Compazine, 102
Compoz, 267, 274. *See also* Over-the-counter drugs
Conference on Evaluation of Muta-genicity of Drugs and Other Chemical Agents, 146
Congress. *See* individual Representa-tives and Senators
Congressional committees, 305–6. *See also* House committees, Senate committees
Congressional Quarterly, 127
Connoisseur foods, 191
Consolidated Royal's Castile Shampoo, 257
Consumer
action, 17 ff., 24, 293 ff., 304–7
and "benefit to risk" ration, 31
-ism, 42–43
protection, and food industry, 161
Consumer Affairs for New York City, 285
"Consumer protectionism," industry's attack on, 173–74
Consumer Reports, 251
Consumer Research Institute, 34
Consumer Safety Administration, 303
Consumer Subcommittee of the Com-mittee on Commerce, House, 305
Contegran, 80

and amphetamines and diet pills, 274–75
budget, 22, 63, 247, 301
Bureau of the Budget, 23, 25
Bureau of Drugs, 125, 133
Bureau of Product Safety, 34
and consumer protection, 17–27
and cosmetic industry, 46, 246–66
and cyclamate ban, 149–61
"Dear Doctor" letters, 116–18
Division of Drug Advertising, 125–26, 132
Division of New Drugs, 80
drug advertising, 103–5, 130–34
and Drug Efficacy Study, 135–47
drug industry, 297 ff.
drug testing, 115
and electric muscle stimulators, 227
food
  industry, and GRAS list, 148–65, 166–87
  poisoning and contamination, 196–200
and herbicides, 216–20
and hexachlorophene, 44–45, 257–66
household hazards, 226 ff.
and mercury poisoning, 206, 208–9
and MER/29, 82–91
and oral contraceptives, 118–30
and over-the-counter drugs, 269 ff., 291
and Panalba case, Upjohn's, 91–97
and Parke-Davis Chloromycetin, 64–78
and prescription drugs, 46–47
Relaxacisor warning, 226
saccharin, 161–64
Shell's No-Pest Strips, 213–15
SKF's stelazine, 105
Spice of Life, 59
staff size, and responsibilities, 22–23, 301–2
and stilbestrol residues in meat, 59–63
thalidomide tragedy, prevention of, in U.S., 79–82
and Vampire blood, 41–42
Food and Drug Law Institute, 36
Food Chemical News, 34, 37
Food, Drug and Cosmetic Act (1938), 25, 47, 60, 261
  1962 amendments to, 79, 81
Food Protection Act of 1972, 291–92
Foil icicles, lead content of, 287
Folic acid, 174
Foster, E. M., 198
Fountain, L. H., 27, 63, 91–93, 97, 123–25, 128. *See also* House Intergovernmental Relations Subcommittee of the Committee on Government Operations
Frankfurters, additives in, 285–86
Freedman, Dr. Daniel, 99
Freedom of Information Act, 53
Free enterprise, big business and, 303–4
Freon, poisoning, 244
Fresca, 149
Freyhan, Dr. Fritz, 102
Friedman, Paul, 153–55

Fritz, Dodge and Olcott, and manufacture of food additives, 36
Fryer, Jerome, 236
Fugate, Scott, 238
Fungicides, mercury-based, 204. *See also* Mercury poisoning
F. W. Woolworth Musical Merry-G-Round Canelon, 32

Gardner, Dr. Elmer, 269–70
G. D. Searle & Company, 121–26
G-11, 262, 265. *See also* Hexachlorophene
General Electric
  and industrial pollution, 207
  and television X-ray leakage, 240
General Fire Extinguishing Company, 224
General Foods, 39
General Mills, 35, 175
General Motors, 42
Generic drugs, vs. brand-name, 21, 58, 109, 140–41, 271, 272, 299
Genetic changes. *See also* Mutations
  additives and, 170, 179–80
  and drugs, 145–46
George Washington University, 172
  School of Medicine, 267
Georgia Pacific, and industrial pollution, 205
Gerber baby foods, additives and, 172
Geritol, 276–78
Germany, thalidomide crisis in, 79–81. *See also* Thalidomide
Gevramet Geriatric Elixir, 32
Gillette's The Hot One Self Heating Shave Cream, dangers of, 254–55
Givaudan Corporation, 265
Glick, William, 206–7
Glutethimide (Doriden), 109
Goddard, Dr. James, 72
Goldberg, Dr. D. C., 126, 134
Gold Seal's Mr. Bubble, irritation to children, 256
Gonyaulax cantenella, in clams, 18
Goodrich, William, 93
Gordon, Ben, 99, 268
Gout, in children, 38
Grant, Bess Myerson, 285–86
GRAS (Generally Recognized as Safe) list, 35, 36–37
  and food industry, 148–65
  National Academy of Sciences review of, 167–87
Gray, Donald, 92–93, 97
"Gray syndrome," 38
Great American Dream Machine, 47–49, 168
Great Atlantic and Pacific Tea Company, 22, 33
Great Britain
  ban on PCB, 194
  drug labeling laws in, 78
  drug pretesting in, 80
  fire hazard deaths in, 238
Greenfield Crab Grass Broadleaf Weed Killer, 218
Gristedes Food Stores, 191

Grocery Manufacturers of America, 36, 149
Gulf Oil Company, 34

Hair dyes, carcinogens in, 247
Hair sprays, and aerosol poisoning, 244, 245 n.
Hansberry, Dr. T. Roy, 214–15
"Hard" pesticides, 215–16
Hart, Philip A., 63, 210, 217, 305
Harvard Medical
  School, 179
  Services, 296
Hasbro Industries, 31–32, 236
Hawaiian Punch recall, 46
Hawk, Robert, 262
Hays, Dr. Harry, 212, 214
Hazardous Substances Act, 236
Hazel Bishop Sudden Change, 251
Head and Shoulders dandruff shampoo, 257
Health and reducing gadgets, 226–27
Heinz Nutritional Research Laboratory, 174
Hemochromatosis, 37
Henry Ford Hospital (Detroit), 54
Herbicides, 18, 24, 34
  poisoning, 219–21
  2, 4-D, 44
  2, 4, 5-T, 44, 216–18
  use of, in Vietnam, 219
Hercules
  and herbicides, manufacture of, 216, 218–21
  and industrial pollution, 205
Heroin, 110
Hertz, Dr. Roy, 127
Hewitt, Dr. William, 136
Hexachlorophene, 43–45, 221
  FDA ban on, 257–66, 288–90
Hickory Farms Foods, 191
Hill, Dr. Henry, 238
Hi-Q Orange Soda recall, 46
H. J. Heinz Company, 163
  additives, and baby foods, 172
Hoffman-LaRoche, 117, 136, 144, 286
Holiday Fair, Inc., Moody Doll, 32
Hollister, Dr. Leon, 100, 106, 108, 109, 111
Holly Farms, 193
Honey Bear Farms, 191
Hooks, Dr. H. A., 71
Hormel's Genoa Salami, 194
Hormone cream, safety of, 251
Hospital supplies, 300. *See also* Intravenous fluid solutions
Hostess Snack Cakes, 276
Household hazards, 222–45
  poisonings, 229–33
House Intergovernmental Relations Subcommittee of the Committee on Government Operations, 123–25, 128, 130–34, 160–61, 283, 288, 302, 306
House Subcommittee on Public Health, 273
Huber, Mrs. Lorraine, 219
Huckleby, Ernest, 204
Hudnut cosmetics, 298
Human sensitivity, and chemicals, 180
Humphrey, Hubert, 177
Huntley-Brinkley show, 155
Hygrade Foods, 59
Hyperactive children, 100
Hypnotic drugs, 100
  definition, 108–9
Hypoplastic anemia, Chloromycetin as cause of, 64–65

Ideal Toy Company, 31, 236
  toy balloon, 234
Imagineering, Inc., 41
Imipramine, 286
"Imminent hazard," 39, 93–95
Industrial pollution, 201–21
Industry. *See also* Drug industry, Food
  and consumerism, 42–43
  bad publicity, effect of, on, 39
  lobbyists, 27, 63, 302
  and product safety, 34
  and public safety, lack of regard for, 21
  self-regulation, attempts at, 21, 44, 50, 61, 172, 232
Insecticides, 18. *See also* Pesticides
Inter-Industry Committee on Aerosol Use, 245
International Minerals and Chemical Corporation, 173–74
Intravenous fluid solutions, Abbott Pharmaceutical's contaminated, 50–58
Iraq, mercury poisoning in, 203
Irma Shorell Contour/35, 250–51
Iron. *See also* Geritol
  deficiency anemia, 277
  fortification, 37
  tablets, 38
Ismelin, 117
Italy
  ban on U.S. metals, 59, 60, 61, 62
  drug labeling laws in, 78
Ivory Flakes, 243

Jacobsen, Dr. Cecil, 170
Japan
  drug labeling laws in, 78
  fire hazard deaths in, 238
  mercury poisoning in, 202–3, 207
  PCB deaths in, 194
J. B. Williams Company, 273, 275, 277
Jeffrey Martin Laboratories, 274
Jennings, Dr. John, 160
Jensen, Malcolm W., 33–34
Jequirity beans, poisonous, 30, 235
Johns Hopkins
  Contraceptive Clinic, 127
  School of Medicine, 282
Johnson, Charles C., 23
Johnson, Nicholas, 283–84
Johnson & Johnson, 30, 33, 116, 135
  feminine hygiene sprays, 264
  First Aid Cream, 221, 258
  Micrin mouthwash, 252
Journal of the American Medical Association, 21, 69, 105, 106
Journal of Law and Economics, 114

Kaiser Industries, and industrial pollution, 205